CELBAN WRITING PREPARATION GUIDE

Healer, Master the CELBAN

Written by Kim Kara M.Ed.
Created for CELBANPrep University
Published by CELBANPrep Publishing

UNDERSTAND THE ROLE OF THE CELBAN

in preparing to become a nurse in Canada

CELBAN WRITING

HOW TO INCREASE YOUR SCORE NOW SO THAT YOU CAN STOP WASTING TIME AND MONEY TAKING ENDLESS COURSES AND FAILING THE TEST OVER AND OVER AGAIN.

What You Will Learn:

- Everything you need to know about the **new CELBAN Writing**.
- What you need to get a high score on both **Task 1** and **Task 2** of CELBAN Writing.
- Tips and topics, **samples and examples**, written by Internationally Educated Nurses like you.
- Get all the examples and answers you need to **increase your score**, to practice **persuasive writing, controversial topics, position pieces,**
- and more...

There are 2 ways to use this guide

1. **Self-Study:** use the lessons and assignments in the textbook, and
2. **During a course:** the 90 Day Challenge at CELBANPrep University.

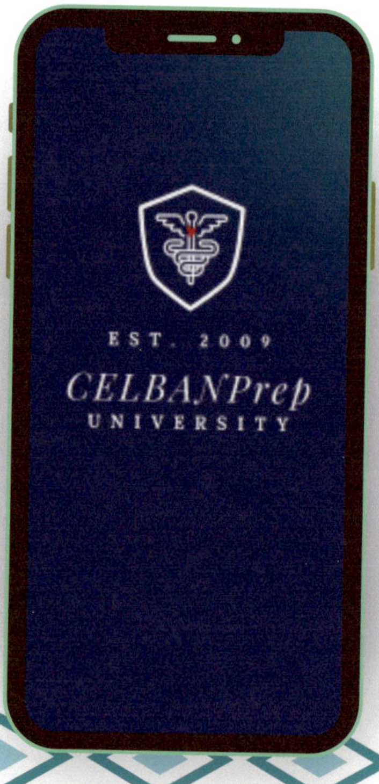

KEYWORDS: CELBAN, writing, examples, samples, tips, videos, topics, questions, practice, persuasive writing, editorials, position pieces, Task 1, Task 2, incident reports, assessment reports, moderately demanding medical situations, comprehend instructions, interact with others, give instructions, get things done.

CELBAN WRITING

COPYRIGHT

Design and Layout by Kim Kara
Visit my website at www.CELBANPrep.ca
Created in Canada
ISBN 978-1-927448-37-3

First Printing: September 2021

CELBAN WRITING

DISCLAIMER

The clinical scenarios described in this book are entirely fictional.
No resemblance to real people or actual cases is intended.
Every effort was made to ensure the accuracy of the material presented in this book at the time of first publication.

Given the policies, procedures and instructions can change at any time, candidates should always read and follow the directions provided on the website at https://www.celbancentre.ca. Candidates use the information, materials and suggestions in this book, and associated resources, at their own risk. Neither Kim Kara nor CELBANPrep assumes any responsibility for candidates' performance on the Canadian English Language Benchmark Assessment for Nurses or any other exam.

CELBANPrep and Kim Kara have no responsibility for the persistence or accuracy of URLs for external or third-party Internet Web sites referred to in this publication and does not guarantee that any content on such Web sites is, or will remain, accurate or appropriate. Information regarding factual information given in this work are correct at the time of publishing. CELBANPrep does not guarantee the accuracy of such information thereafter.

CELBAN WRITING

ABOUT CELBANPREP

- Are you a motivated Internationally Educated Health Professional?
- Are you seeking licensure to practice in Canada?
- Are you preparing for an English Proficiency exam:
    - CELBAN, or
    - IELTS.

Are you looking for ways to prepare for your exam in less time, with less stress, and more wellness - explore CELBANPrep University at www.celbanprep.ca!

OUR MISSION

▶ We create affordable and accessible resources for Internationally Educated Health Professionals - Internationally Educated Nurses, Doctors, Physiotherapists, X-Ray Technicians, Midwives, International Medical Graduates and more -> that are:

✓ preparing for English Proficiency Exams by
✓ focusing on professional development in Canada.

OUR CLASSROOM APP

▶ We provide CELBAN Information, CELBAN Material and CELBAN Preparation courses that are accessible on your Android or iOS phones or tablets. There is also an app for Chromebooks.

CELBAN WRITING

HOW WE DO THIS

Since the beginning of time, back in 2009, when I, Kim Kara, started creating resources for Internationally Educated Health Professionals preparing for the CELBAN exam, nothing was available. I worked for an employment centre. My nurses would come to me asking for books to prepare for the CELBAN and there were none. So, I got a second contract and started creating CELBAN preparation material.
It didn't take me long to realize that it wasn't enough just to create a book or to create a website.

CELBAN ONLINE

I had to create so much more; I needed to create so many different things:

- **CELBAN online courses**: textbooks, workbooks, lesson plans.
- **CELBAN online classes**: small groups that get together on a regular basis to practice skills taught during the online courses.
- **CELBAN material**: quizzes, handouts, assignments to practice skills required to pass the CELBAN.
- **CELBAN reviewers**: e-books, websites, blog posts, Facebook updates that expose IENs to the format and structure - expectations - of the CELBAN.
- **CELBAN intensives**: CELBAN online courses, classes and material that helps people to decrease the amount of time it takes to prepare for the CELBAN.

THREE OPTIONS

- **Study alone, l**east expensive, exploring the reviewers.
- **Subscribe to the CELBANPrep University**: to get access to more material, Master Classes, and quizzes, Or
- **Enroll at CELBANPrep University** to complete a course or take a class.

CELBAN WRITING

ABOUT CELBANPREP WRITING

Since the beginning of time, back in 2009, I started preparing Internationally Educated Nurses for the CELBAN exam.
I started with 6 nurses in a library at the employment agency I was working at. I created the lessons, and I saw them struggle.

- They didn't know where to start for the writing task.
- They didn't know how to organize their thinking.
- They didn't know how to manage their time.

That is why I created CELBANPrep Writing Level One, encouraging IENs to write about their life, their family, their experiences. What was wonderful was that with the changes to CELBAN Writing in 2018, I had already created a CELBAN online course for Writing Task 1: CELBANPrep Writing Level One!

So, if you are wondering if CELBANPrep Writing is still relevant with the changes to CELBAN Writing in 2018: the answer is, "YES!"

CELBANPrep Writing Level One teaches you skills:

- you can apply to any exam including the CELBAN, the IELTS, the CELPIP (for Immigration).
- you can apply to both tasks including CELBAN Writing Task 1 and Task 2.
- that will impact your career as a whole: not just help you prepare for the exam!

CELBANPrep Writing Level Two teaches you how to apply these skills when you write in a medical context: incident reports, etc.
Learn more about how to prepare for CELBAN Writing through CELBANPrep University!

CELBAN WRITING PREPARATION GUIDE

Healers Heal: They Don't Steal.

If you, or someone you know, has not paid for this book, you may be an accessory to a crime. It is a criminal offense to steal - to make and distribute photocopies or digital scans - of published works without the permission of the author or publisher.

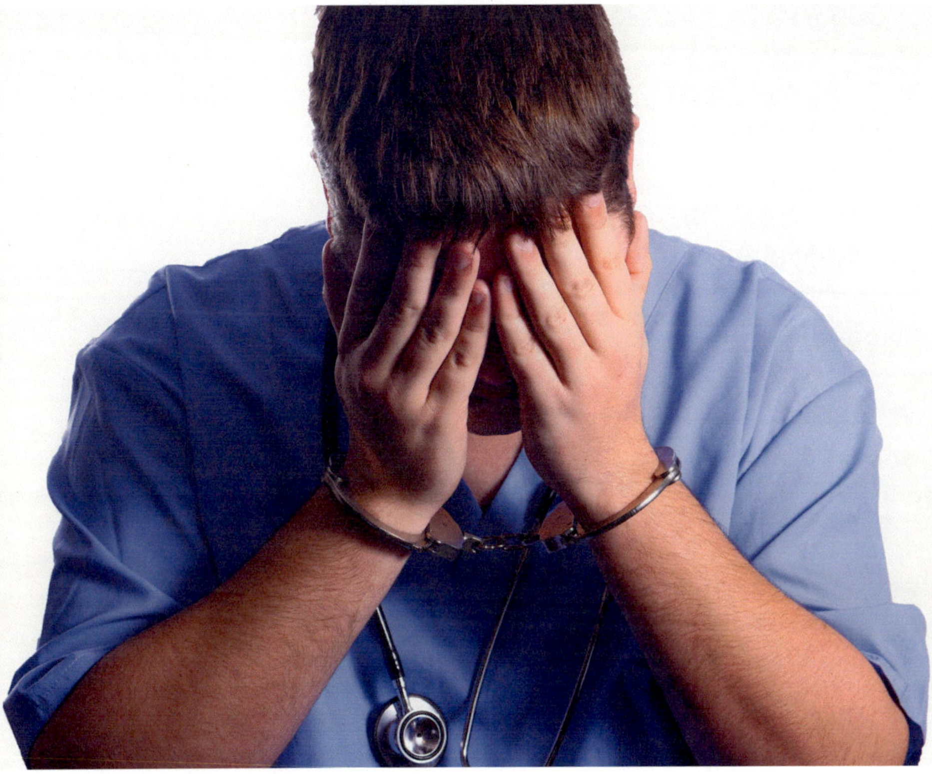

UNDERSTAND COPYRIGHT LAWS

The only reason why CELBANPrep exists is because IENs have invested in their futures through Kim and CELBANPrep. That is why, if this is s stolen copy then you are, in effect, stealing from the future.
Are you a healer who heals, or a healer who steals?

CELBAN WRITING

TABLE OF CONTENTS

THREE OPTIONS

1. **Study alone,** least expensive, exploring the prep guides and reviewers.
2. **Subscribe to the CELBANPrep University:** to get access to more material, Master Classes, and quizzes, Or
3. **Enroll at CELBANPrep University** to complete a course or take a class.

CELBAN WRITING PREPARATION GUIDE

Healer, Know Thy Self

Created by CELBANPrep University
Published by CELBANPrep Publishing

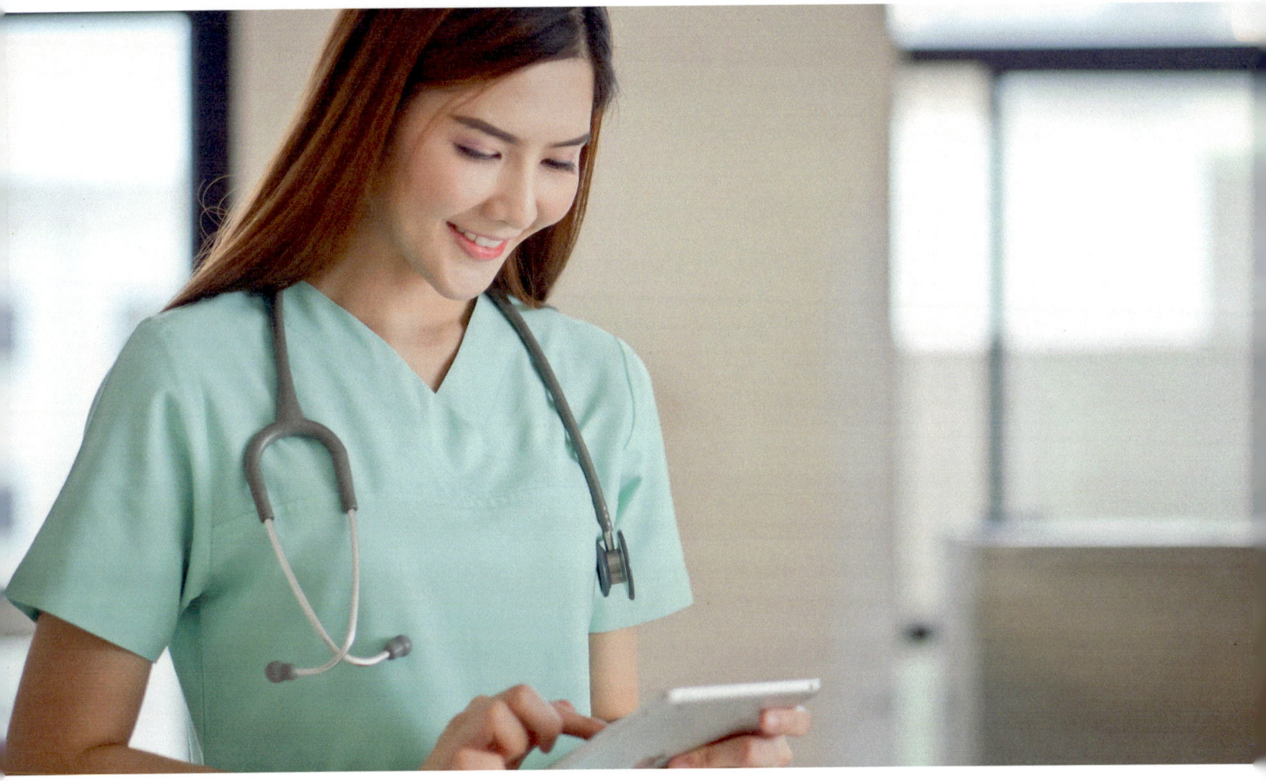

UNDERSTAND THE ROLE OF THE CELBAN

By contemplating your role as a nurse

CELBAN WRITING

UNDERSTANDING THE CELBAN

When you sit for the CELBAN exam, there are four "Competencies" or contexts you will be asked about. The exam has been created to determine how well you create communication, in the English language, when you are:

1 Interacting with Others

2 Intrepreting/Giving Instructions

3 Getting Things Done

4 Comprehending Information

That is why the first part of this Writing Preparation Guide starts by asking you to think about who you are and what you do as a nurse:

- Why you became a nurse, and who your role models are, and
- What happens, when as a nurse, what you write is misunderstood?

The implicit reason for the design of this section is so that you can determine what skills you, as an individual, need to improve upon so that you can get the required score on the CELBAN and to achieve your dreams of life in Canada.

REFERENCE: Canadian Language Benchmarks:
English as a second language for adults
by the CCLB

CELBAN WRITING

WHAT YOU WILL LEARN IN THIS SECTION

There are three competencies you will be developing and addressing in this section:

1 Interacting with Others

2 Intrepreting/ Giving Instructions

3 Comprehending Information

Interacting with Others:

- In order to interact with others you need to know your self, and be able to communicate things about your self with ease.
- It is also important, on the CELBAN, that you are able to write in both a formal and a non-formal context.
- Through your writing, the assessors will be paying attention to your tone, your vocabulary, and how you write, to determine if you can modify how you write based on who you are writing to.

Interpreting Instructions:

- Both the CELBAN and this guide are created with specific instructions to see if you will not only follow the instructions, but follow them in order.

Comprehending Information:

- The format of this guide is to present information about the CELBAN, so that you understand that the structure and intent is different from the IELTS. Thus, it is important to prepare for this exam in new and maybe even uncomfortable ways (at first).

NAME ______________________ **DATE** ______________________

CELBAN WRITING

HEALER KNOW THY SELF

Write down all the reasons why you became a nurse. Remember to include your mental, emotional, spiritual, social, cultural and financial reasons. You may choose whether to write your answers **in paragraph form or point form.**

NAME ______________________ **DATE** ______________________

CELBAN WRITING

HEALER KNOW THY SELF

Contemplate the ROLE of a Nurse.
Think about all the different roles you play, as a nurse, with all the different contexts. **Write down a point-form list** of all the different times and situation that you use writing to communicate thoughts, ideas, encouragement and feelings. Include both formal and non-formal situations: with patients, with colleagues,
and with supervisors.

NAME ______________________ **DATE** ______________________

______________________ ______________________

CELBAN WRITING

HEALER KNOW THY SELF

Contemplate the ROLE of a Nurse.
Contemplate, think about, and remember the times when, as a nurse, what you have written was/could be misunderstood. **Briefly write about your experiences. What happened?**
What could happen? What were the consequences?
What might the consequences be?

NAME ______________________ **DATE** ______________________

CELBAN WRITING

HEALER KNOW THY SELF

Contemplate the ROLE of a Nurse.
Considering all of the different times and situations that you, as a nurse, are required to write thoughts, feelings, hopes, and even encouragement. Would you say that those situations were: not demanding, moderately demanding, or demanding.
Choose your answer and explain why, in paragraph form.

NAME ____________________ **DATE** ____________________

CELBAN WRITING

HEALER KNOW THY SELF

Conclusion

Which writing skills do you need to develop so that you can writing competently - in English- in moderately demanding situations as a nurse, in Canada? **Create a point-form list.**

NAME ______________________ **DATE** ______________________

CELBAN WRITING

HEALER KNOW THY SELF

Conclusion

Using the list of skills you need to acquire: **create a list of questions** you can ask prospective teachers, mentors and guides (review centres and service providers) to discern and determine if that individual or organization can help you to prepare for the CELBAN.

CELBAN WRITING

UNDERSTANDING THE CELBAN

That is why the required score on CELBAN Writing is what it is. The decision of the score has been made - individually and collectively - by the provincial licensing bodies. They determined that as a nurse, when you write, you write in moderately demanding situations, because there are three levels when it comes to scores for the CLB/CELBAN:

1. Beginner: non-demanding
   - scores 1-4
2. Intermediate: moderately demanding
   - scores 5-8
3. Advanced: demanding
   - scores 9-12

What that means, is that to get the required score in Writing on the CELBAN you must be able to interact with others, follow instructions, get things done, and understand information in moderately demanding situations.

Q. What skills do you have, and which do you need to develop?
A. We will explore that in the next section.

***REFERENCE: Canadian Language Benchmarks: English as a second language for adults* by the CCLB**

CELBAN WRITING

UNDERSTANDING THE CELBAN

What you need to understand, in going into the CELBAN, is that it is not the IELTS. In fact the CELBAN is unlike any other English exam. Where the IELTS was created in the UK for all professions, the CELBAN was created in Canada for nurses. That is why it is important to remember what the C and the N in CELBAN stand for:

C anadian
E nglish
L anguage
B enchmark
A ssessment
N urses

For those reasons, **IT IS NOT POSSIBLE to prepare for the CELBAN the same way you would for the IELTS. Why?**

Because *the CELBAN was created as a gateway into your professional life in Canada.* It is about ensuring you have the qualifications of both creating and interpreting professional communications clearly and accurately in moderately demanding to demanding situations when it comes to: interacting with others, giving/understanding instructions, getting things done, and understanding information.

CELBAN WRITING

CHAPTER REVIEW: CHECKING UNDERSTANDING

What are the 4 competencies being evaluated on the CELBAN?

How many levels are there, on the CELBAN, what are they?

What is the required score on CELBAN Writing? Why? What does it mean when you get this score?

CELBAN WRITING PREPARATION GUIDE

Healer, Know Thy Self

Created by CELBANPrep University
Published by CELBANPrep Publishing

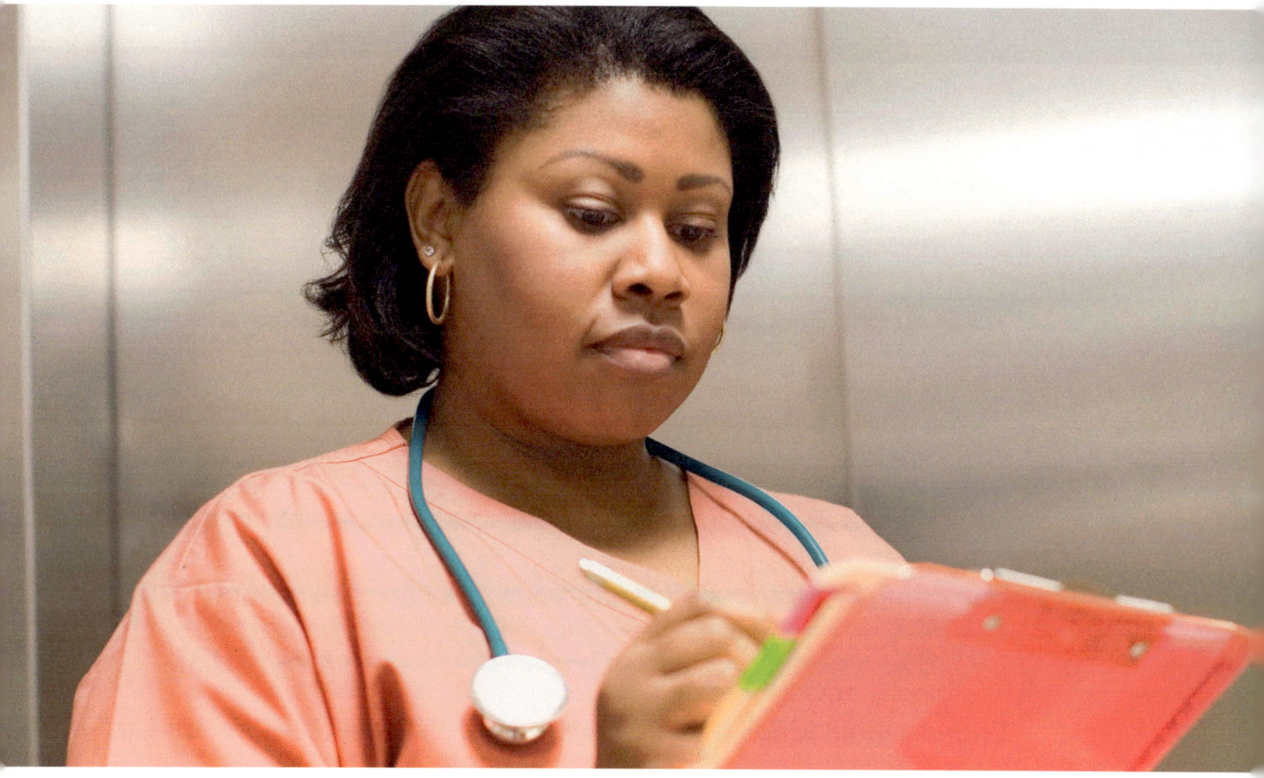

SKILL DEVELOPMENT AND THE CELBAN

Understanding the Skills you MUST demonstrate as a nurse in Canada

CELBAN WRITING

SELF-EVALUATION

Evaluate Your Skill Level
INSTRUCTIONS: Use the following scale to determine how well you do the following in English:

Communicate, in writing, in professional/formal contexts.

0% ________________________________ 100%

Communicate, in writing, in professional/informal contexts.

0% ________________________________ 100%

Write clearly and accurately in moderately demanding situations.

0% ________________________________ 100%

Communicate both implicit and explicit meanings, in writing.

0% ________________________________ 100%

Use complex stentence structures, with only a few errors.

0% ________________________________ 100%

Express main ideas with supporting details, examples, or stories.

0% ________________________________ 100%

INSTRUCTIONS: How often do you do the following:

Spell correctly?

0% ——— 100%

Use punctuation correctly?

0% ——— 100%

Capitalize correctly? Write numbers, use abbreviations correctly?

0% ——— 100%

Use articles correctly?

0% ——— 100%

Keep your verb tense consistent?

0% ——— 100%

Make agreement errors?

0% ——— 100%

Create coherent pieces of writing?

0% ——— 100%

Use phrases and connectors correctly?

0% ——— 100%

Edit your own work? Correct your mistakes?

0% ——— 100%

INSTRUCTIONS: How well do you do the following:

Interact with others, in writing?

0% ———————————————— 100%

Write persuasively, so that you get things done?

0% ———————————————— 100%

Write in a way that gives clear direction and instructions?

0% ———————————————— 100%

Write in a way that communicates what you understand?

0% ———————————————— 100%

What have you learned about your self when it comes to writing in English?

CELBAN WRITING

PRIORITIZING SKILL DEVELOPMENT

INSTRUCTIONS:

Use your answers to rank the skills on the previous page as:

- Urgent & Important to develop because it is a weakness that is negatively impacting your life, your career, and your score;
- Not Urgent but Important to develop;
- Urgent but Important to develop; or
- Neither Urgent nor Important to develop because the skill is a strength.

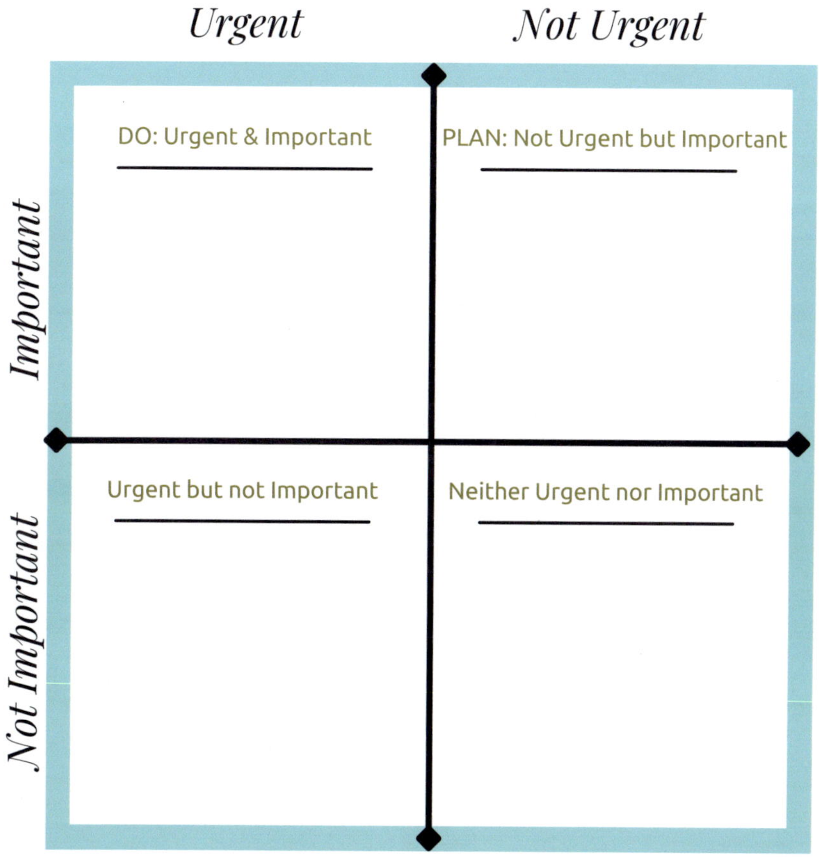

CELBAN WRITING PREPARATION GUIDE

Healer, Decide for Your Self

Created by CELBANPrep University
Published by CELBANPrep Publishing

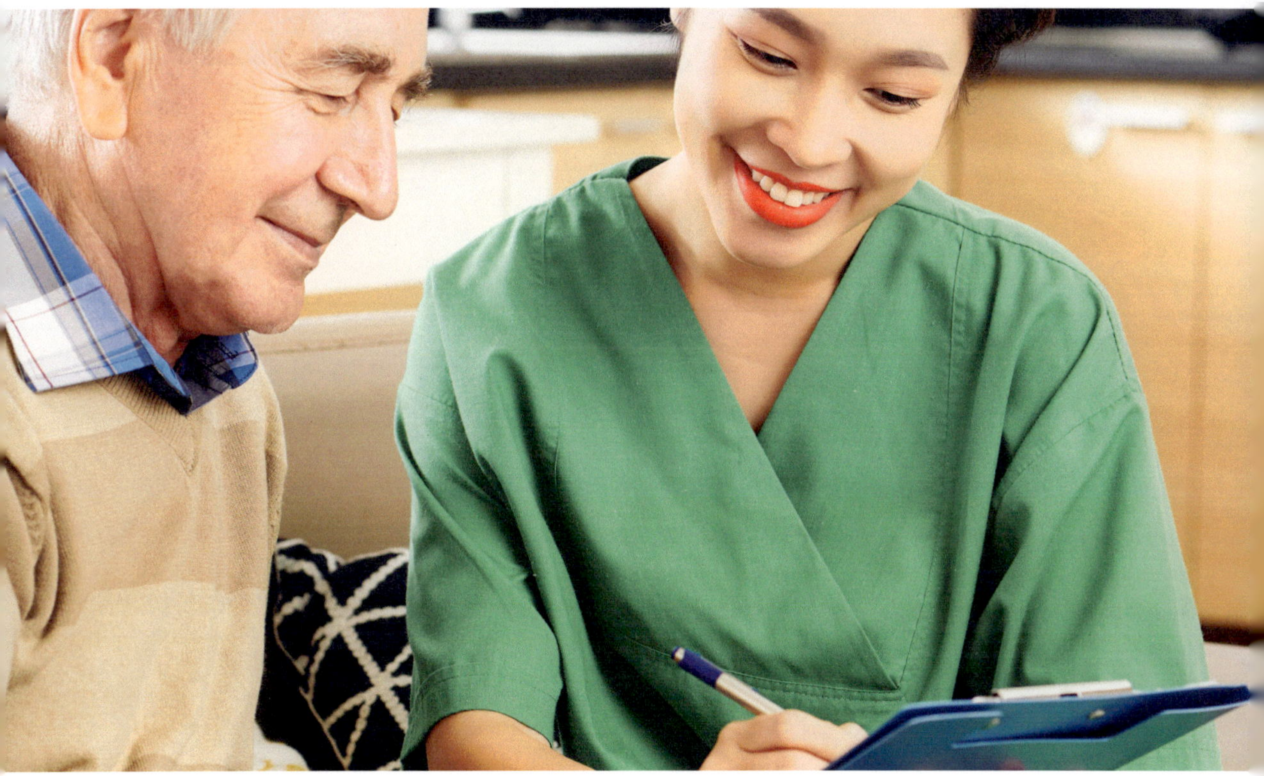

SKILL DEVELOPMENT AND THE CELBAN

Getting Things Done by Exploring Your Options

CELBAN WRITING

REFLECTIVE ACTIVITY

INSTRUCTIONS: Use this page to brainstorm all the ways you have prepared for the writing portion of your English proficiency exams, like the CELBAN and IELTS, in the past.

- Include the different kinds of resources, material, activities that you have engaged in.

NOTE: Ensure that you have included: online resources or face to face, group work, live sessions, videos, worksheets, having your work reviewed, being encouraged, being criticized, working alone, working with a partner, large lecture halls... and any other experience you have had as a student and adult learner. When you have exhausted all ideas, follow the instructions below.

INSTRUCTIONS: Use the following legend to colour code how effective the brainstormed methods, listed previously, were in teaching you and helping you to learn how to write, accurately, in a professional context: both formally and informally.

- red -> not effective at all
- yellow -> somewhat effective
- green -> very effective

What have you learned about your self when it comes to learning to write in English? What are your needs? What works best for you?

CELBAN WRITING

OBJECTIVE INQUIRY

Basically there are three ways for us, as learners, to engage with new material. Each has its own pros and cons.

- working alone -> least expensive
- peer mentoring-> somewhat effective
- professional guidance -> very effective

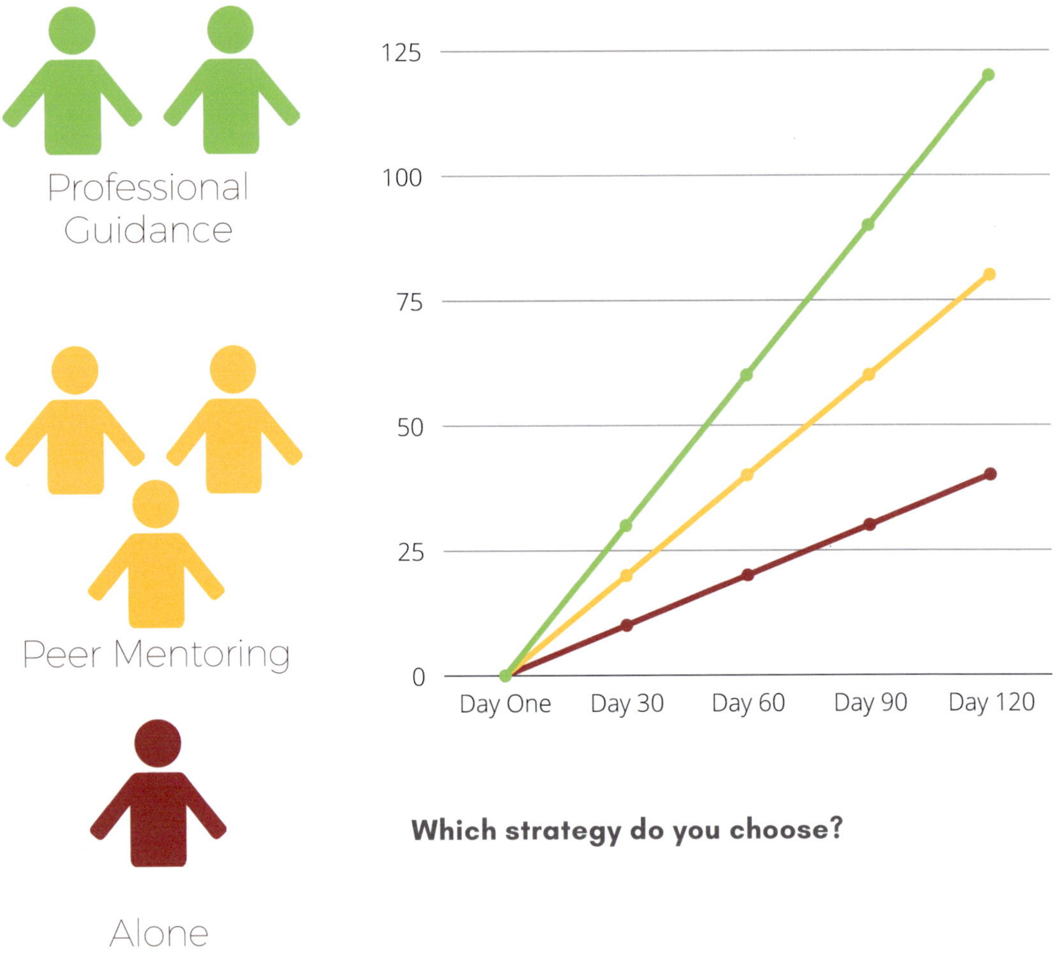

Which strategy do you choose?

Which is the most effective way, and why?

How can what you are learning in this preparation guide save you both time and money?

If you could learn

the

SKILLS

you

MUST

know

to PASS

CELBAN

WRITING,

Would You Be Interested?

CELBAN WRITING

YOUR OPTIONS

Because CELBANPrep has always had a Compassionate Pricing Policy, there are three options available for you to prepare for the CELBAN:

1. Accessing ***CELBAN preparation guides*** available internationally through Amazon.
2. Getting a subscription to ***CELBANPrep University*** for a nominal monthly fee.
3. Enrolling in ***CELBANPrep University's 90 Day Challenge.***

What that means is that you have choices: depending on your budget and what works for you. Of course, the most ideal is attending a class with a qualified teacher. But, the others are available as well, so that you have direction on how to prepare while you save your money so that you can afford CELBANPrep Course.

Q. Which would you choose if money was no object: you didn't have to worry about how much it cost?

www.writing.CELBANPrep.info

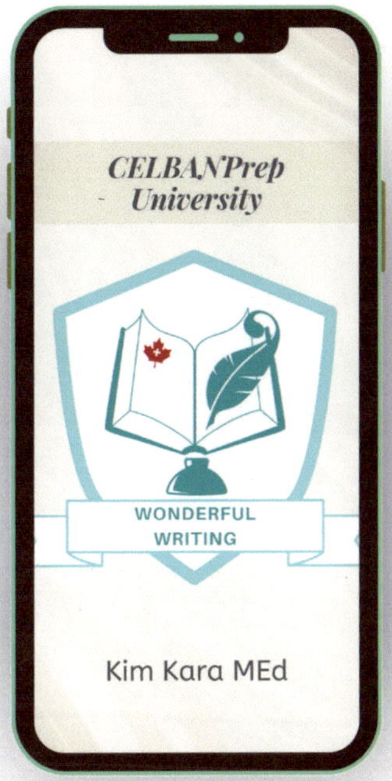

CRAFT YOUR WORDS

MASTER THE ART OF WONDERFUL WRITING

CELBAN WRITING PREPARATION GUIDE

Healer, Prepare Your Self

Created by CELBANPrep University
Published by CELBANPrep Publishing

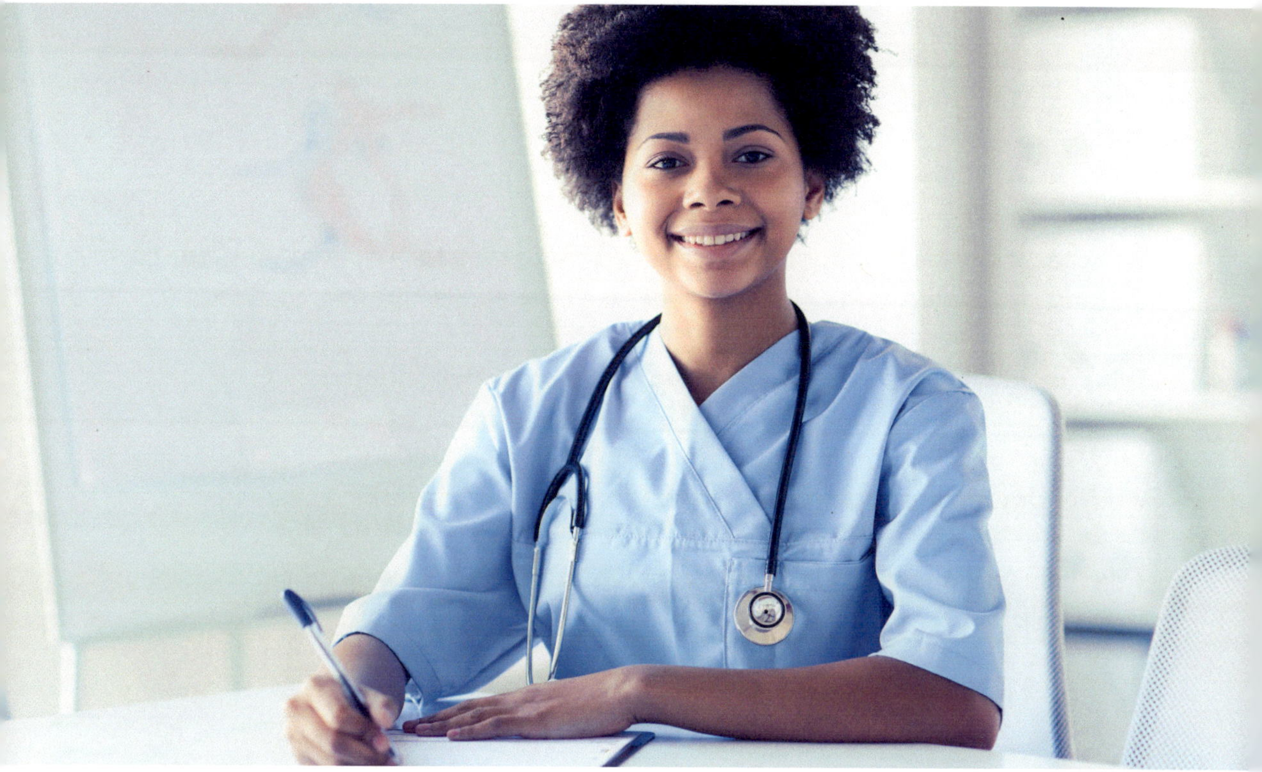

CELBAN WRITING: WRITING ABOUT MEDICAL TOPICS

Getting Things Done and How to Prepare for the CELBAN

CELBAN WRITING

UNDERSTANDING THE CELBAN

Remember, when it comes to the CELBAN, there are four main competencies that you require in life and in your career to achieve success:

1. Interacting with Others
2. Intrepreting/Giving Instructions
3. Getting Things Done
4. Comprehending Information

So, when it comes to preparing for the CELBAN exam, take time to consider the material, resources, and courses or classes you are investigating.

Think about what you need, to develop the skills you identified as:

- Urgent and Important (skills to develop now), and
- Not Urgent, but important (skills to plan to develop next).

Take time to contemplate and consider: "What is the best way for me to develop these skills?"

REFERENCE: Canadian Language Benchmarks: English as a second language for adults by the CCLB

The best way for me to develop these writing skills is...

How to Prepare for the CELBAN WRITING TASKS

as a self-study

CELBAN WRITING

TASKS

Congratulations! You have completed the self-inventory. Now it is time for you to learn more about Task 1 and Task 2 of CELBAN Writing.

By now you know that the CELBAN is unlike any other exam you have taken. You understand that because it is a Canadian exam, and because it is in a nursing context, that there are skills that you MUST demonstrate on the exam to get the required score. You also know that these skills are to be demonstrated in four different contexts: interacting with others, getting things done, giving/understanding instructions, and understanding information. Now you get to see, know and understand how that comes together for Writing Tasks 1 and 2.

At CELBANPrep we often get asked:

- **Can I see writing samples?**
- **What kind of topics are on the CELBAN exam?**

As you can interpret from what you have already experienced in this guide: those questions come from people preparing for the IELTS and not the CELBAN. On the CELBAN they can ask you questions about any medical topic as long as the topic falls into one of the four categories: interacting with others, getting things done, giving/understanding instructions, and understanding information.

That is why it is important to **STOP ASKING FOR SAMPLES AND ABOUT TOPICS, because the CELBAN does not test your knowledge, it tests your skill level.**

CELBAN WRITING

THE FORMAT OF THE EXAM

What do you mean the CELBAN does not test my knowledge, it tests my skills? What does that mean? How do I prepare for an exam like that?

These are very valid questions for people who have been preparing for English exams, like the IELTS, in ways that are not consistent with the Canadian education system, the Canadian medical system.

When it comes to the CELBAN, the Canadian English Language Benchmark Assessment for Nurses, you are being tested on your ability to communicate as a nurse: both creating (writing and speaking) and interpreting communication (reading and listening).

There are FIVE KNOWLEDGES that you are being assessed on:

- Grammar Knowledge,
- Cohesion Knowledge,
- Interpretive Knowledge,
- Emotional Intelligence, and Social Intelligence.

And so they will ask you questions, that allow you to demonstrate those five knowledge bases:

- writing about medical topics, and
- writing in a medical context.

This is important for you to know, should you decide to hire a teacher, tutor or review centre. Use this information to evaluate whether they can teach you these knowledges: especially emotional and social intelligence in a way that is consistent with the Canadian culture. Doing so will save you both time and money.

All TASKS:

- **Grammar Knowledge**
- **Cohesion Knowledge**
- **Interpretive Knowledge**
- **Emotional Intelligence**
- **Social Intelligence**

Skills to be demonstrated:

Create a coherent pieces of writing.

Communicate, in writing, with an appropriate tone and language.

Communicate both implicit and explicit meanings, in writing.

Express main ideas with supporting details, examples, or stories.

Use complex stentence structures, with only a few errors.

Use phrases and connectors correctly.

Spell and capitalize correctly.

Use punctuation correctly.

Use articles correctly.

Keep your verb tense consistent.

Avoid making agreement errors.

Writing about a Medical Issue

- Understanding Information
- Getting Things Done

Skills to be demonstrated:

Create a coherent pieces of writing.

Communicate, in writing, with an appropriate tone and language.

Express main ideas with supporting details, examples, or stories.

Communicate both implicit and explicit meanings, in writing.

Write persuasively, so that you get things done.

If applicable, give clear direction and instructions.

Skill Practice

There are many different writing devices you can use for this task. Writing is a creative activity. It is an expression of your self! Whether it be a letter to the editor, a persuasive piece, giving written instructions, compare and contrasting or engaging in medical education: the intent of this task is to evaluate your ability to get things done, in writing, once you understand information (about something that is common knowledge in your field.) Thus research is not required. ***How you express your thoughts, your ideas, your feelings, your opinions, your experience is what matters.***

CELBAN WRITING

TOPICS

Internationally Educated Nurses often ask questions about CELBAN Writing: writing about medical topics. They want a list of topics.

What they do not understand is that
there is an endless supply of writing samples and topics.

INSTRUCTIONS:

Create a list of medical topics that you can write about and that you can use to practice and demonstrate the skills on the previous page.

CELBAN WRITING

TOPIC SOURCES

There is also an endless supply of sources for medical topics. Current events, tv shows, movies, and the lives of friends and family are filled with controversial medical topics to write about.

INSTRUCTIONS:

Create a list of sources where you could generate your list of medical topics so that you can practice and demonstrate the skills required of you when it comes to CELBAN Writing.

What have you learned about CELBAN Writing: writing about medical topics.

CELBAN WRITING PREPARATION GUIDE

Healer, Communicate Clearly

Created by CELBANPrep University
Published by CELBANPrep Publishing

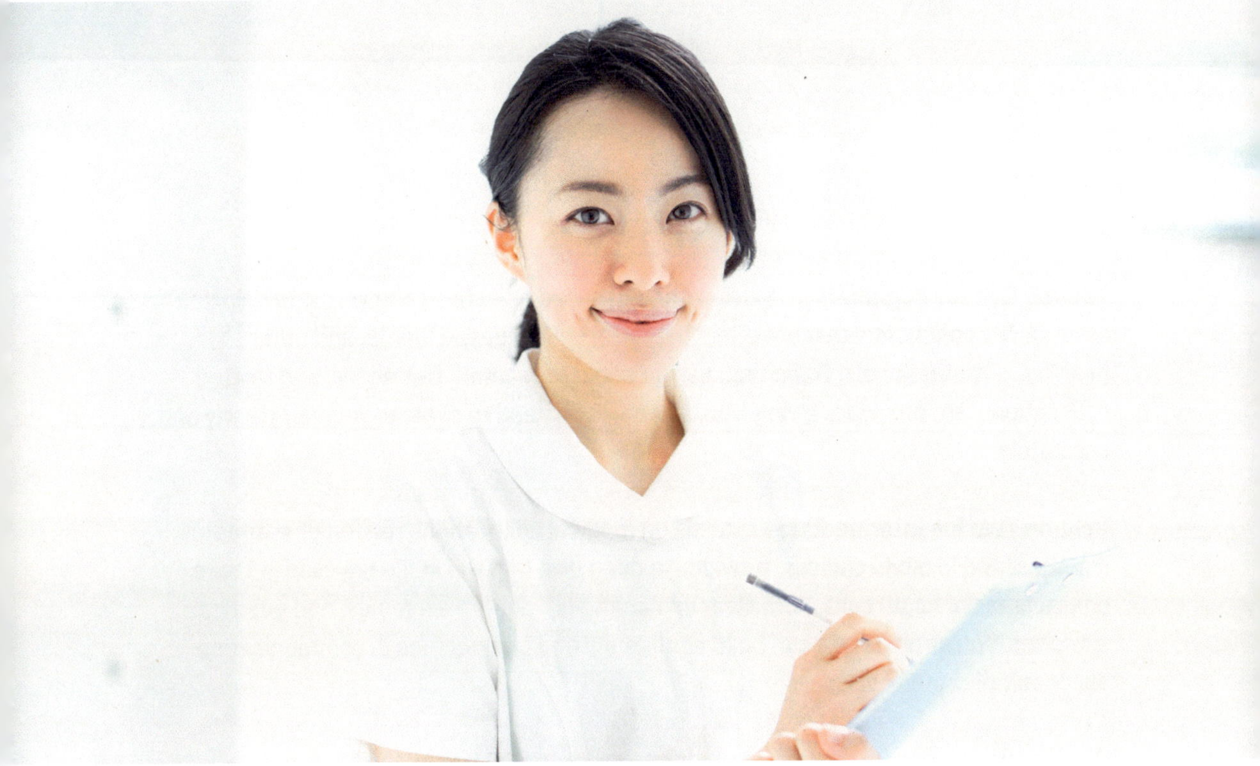

CELBAN WRITING MEDICAL REPORTS

How to Prepare for the CELBAN

Introducing the Medical English Language Mastery Series

Medical Collocations: A Companion to Prefect *Medical Grammar*

Unlock the Power of Precise Communication with the *Medical Collocation Dictionary Series.* Introducing the ultimate language resource for Internationally Educated Healthcare Professionals (IEHPs) looking to improve their communication skills in medical settings! This two-volume medical collocation dictionary provides a comprehensive and easy-to-use guide to the common words and phrases used by healthcare professionals in English-speaking countries.

MEDICAL ENGLISH LANGUAGE MASTERY

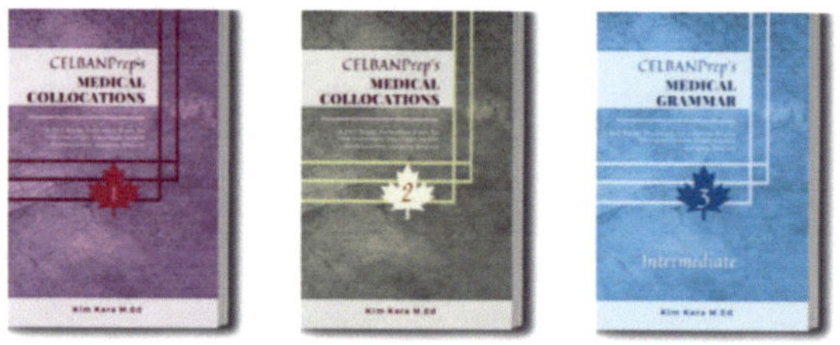

Volume One for Beginners includes commonly used adjectives and verbs, to help you as an IEHPs communicate more effectively with colleagues, patients, and other healthcare professionals. Definition, part of speech, example sentences, and related collocations, are provided, giving you the tools you need to express yourself clearly and accurately.

Volume Two for Intermediates focuses on medical collocations related to symptoms, illnesses, and lifestyle choices, providing a deep dive into the language used in these crucial areas of healthcare. With clear explanations, real-life examples, and practical exercises, you as an IEHPs can build confidence and competence in communicating about complex medical issues.

Whether you're a nurse, doctor, or other healthcare professional, the *Medical Collocation Dictionary* series is the essential resource for mastering the language of medicine and providing the highest quality patient care. **Start communicating with clarity and confidence– order your copy from Amazon today!**

When you read
WRITING
samples
YOU
do not
learn how to
demonstrate skills.
Practice is Required
TO PASS
the CELBAN exam.

All TASKS:

- **Grammar Knowledge**
- **Cohesion Knowledge**
- **Interpretive Knowledge**
- **Emotional Intelligence**
- **Social Intelligence**

Skills to be demonstrated:

Create a coherent pieces of writing.

Communicate, in writing, with an appropriate tone and language.

Communicate both implicit and explicit meanings, in writing.

Express main ideas with supporting details, examples, or stories.

Use complex stentence structures, with only a few errors.

Use phrases and connectors correctly.

Spell and capitalize correctly.

Use punctuation correctly.

Use articles correctly.

Keep your verb tense consistent.

Avoid making agreement errors.

Writing a Medical Report

- Interacting with Others
- Giving/Understanding Instructions

Skills to be demonstrated:

Write in a way that communicates what you understand.

Write clearly and accurately in a moderately demanding situation.

Communicate, in writing, with an appropriate tone and language.

Communicate clear direction and instructions.

Explain a sequence of events clearly and accurately.

Express main ideas with supporting details.

Use appropriate sentence structure, with only a few errors.

Write numbers correctly.

Use abbreviations correctly.

Use medical phrases correctly.

Skill Practice

Traditionally the assessment of an IENs ability to interact with others, and understanding instructions happens through a medical report. We will explore incident reports, and assessment reports.

CELBAN WRITING

SAMPLES OF MEDICAL REPORTS

Internationally Educated Nurses often ask for: writing samples for CELBAN Writing, for medical reports.

What they do not understand is that there is an endless amount of writing samples and topics.

INSTRUCTIONS:

Create a list of sources where you can get writing samples. We started the list for you.

But remember, simply reading samples will not teach you the skills you are required to demonstrate on the CELBAN exam. First, you must decide, practice, and overcome to achieve.

- this guide,
- the Dear Kim blog (www.dear-kim.com) search "report",
- the CELBANPrep University app,
- CELBANPrep's 90 Day Challenge, and
- medical documentation textbooks (US and Canada)

CELBAN WRITING

REPORT TOPICS

There is also an endless supply of topic ideas for medical reports. Experience, tv shows, movies, and the lives of friends and family are filled with patient histories and incidents that you can write about.

INSTRUCTIONS:

Create a list of incidents and brief patient descriptions that you can write about as a medical report.

What have you learned about CELBAN Writing: medical reports.

CELBAN WRITING

TIPS & TRICKS

Do you watch medical TV shows, movies or documentaries?

- What do you do? Do you simply watch them passively, or do you engage more actively?

Writing about Medical Topics Task

- Imagine ways to engage more fully actively in what you are watching.
- When you are watching a documentary or something about current events or medical topics:
  - Determine your opinion. Articulate your thoughts, feelings, and opinions about the topic. Practice communicating YOUR perspective both in writing and speaking.
  - Then edit your writing for grammar, punctuation cohesion, and sentence structure.

Writing Medical Reports

- Imagine ways to engage in movies and TV shows as if you are present in the scenario.
  - If an incident happens: write a report.
  - When an ambulance arrives, what do the Emergency Medical Technicians report?
  - If a patient is admitted, write out a medical history report.
  - When doctors, or other health professionals, are providing instructions: document what happens. Pay attention to the sequence of events.
  - Then edit your writing for grammar, punctuation cohesion, and sentence structure.

CELBAN WRITING PREPARATION GUIDE

Healer, Discover More

Created by CELBANPrep University
Published by CELBANPrep Publishing

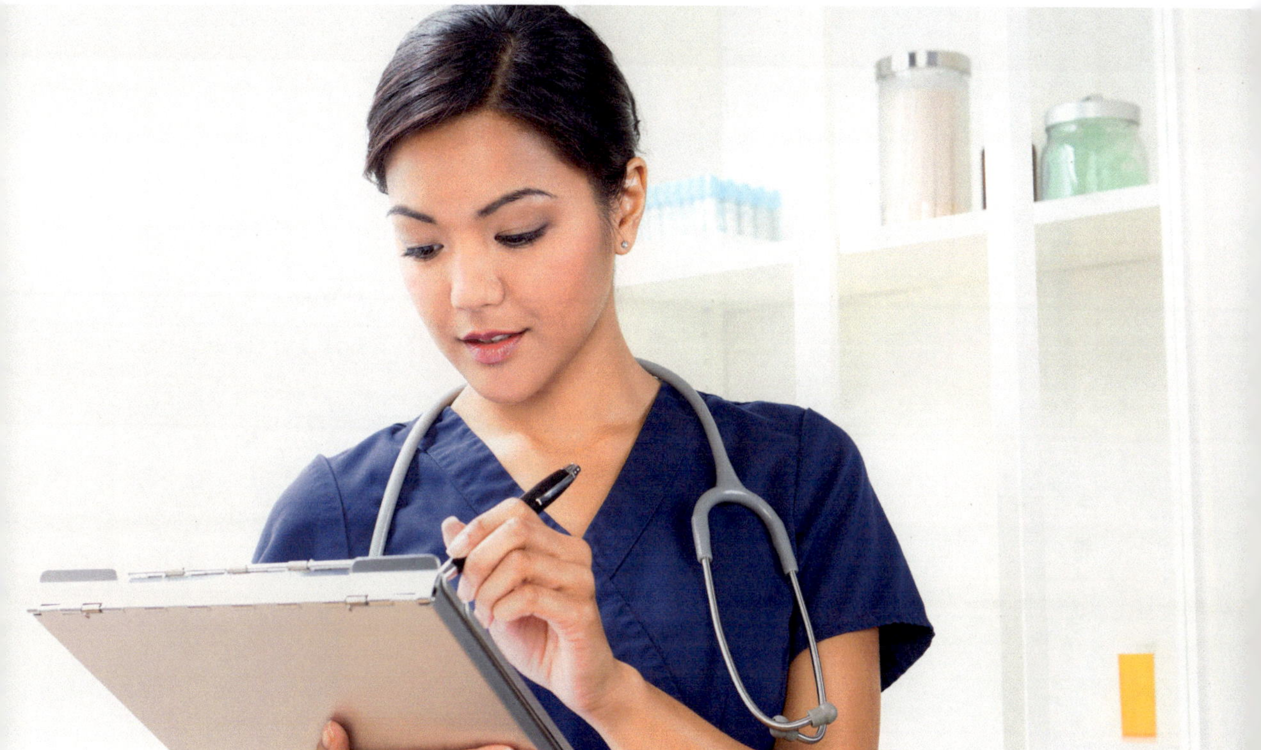

CELBAN WRITING TASK 1 & 2

How to Prepare for the CELBAN

CELBAN WRITING

A YEAR IN PEXELS

Example

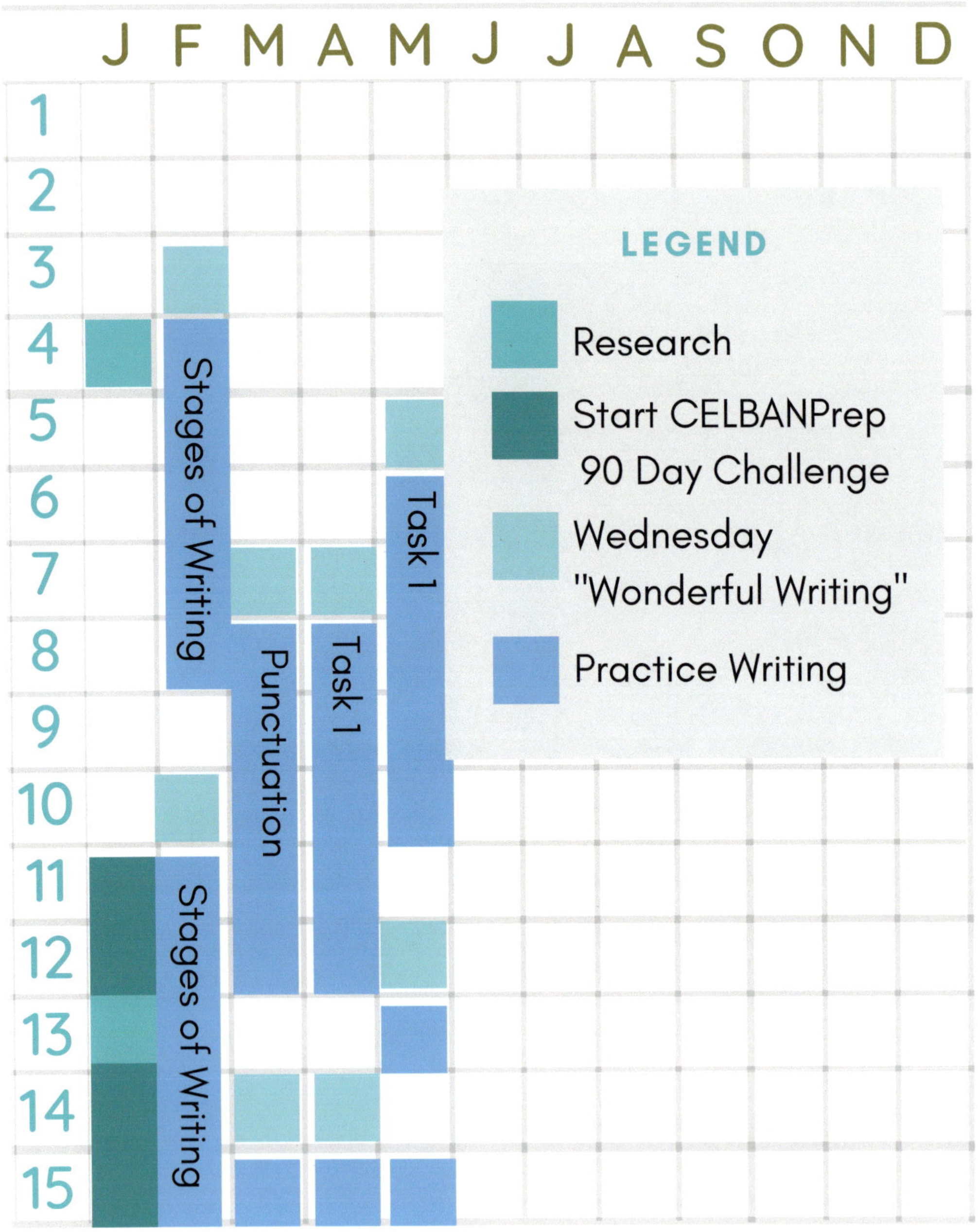

CELBAN WRITING

A YEAR IN PEXELS

Do you need ways to stay motivated?

- Do you get distracted?
- It is difficult to see your improvements?
- Do you struggle with finding time or energy to prepare for the CELBAN?

A Year in Pexels

Using pixels has become a popular way of tracking habits, events, activities and moods. Use the following pages to track your preparation for CELBAN writing.

How it works

There are several ways for you to use pixels. When you use this organizational study tool in combination with the STUDY PLANNERS available through CELBANPrep University, you can keep track of:

- how much time you spent studying each day/week/month.
- which CELBAN Grammar Intensive module you are working on. Nouns & Articles? Verbs & Verbals? Agreement? Punctuation?
- which task you have practiced. Task 1? Writing about medical topics? Task 2? Writing in a medical context?
- which knowledge base you focused on. Is it grammar, cohesion, interpretive abilities, social intelligence, or emotional intelligence.

CELBAN WRITING

A YEAR IN PEXELS

Keep track of how frequently you practice your writing: Task 1 & 2.

	J	F	M	A	M	J	J	A	S	O	N	D
1												
2												
3												
4												
5												
6												
7												
8												
9												
10												
11												
12												
13												
14												
15												

INSTRUCTIONS:

- Create a colour coding system.
- Use numbers
- Document your progress daily, by filling in the box for the day.
- Then, write about how you feel about your progress.

	J	F	M	A	M	J	J	A	S	O	N	D
16												
17												
18												
19												
20												
21												
22												
23												
24												
25												
26												
27												
28												
29												
30												

CELBAN WRITING

ONE YEAR STUDY TRACKER

	1	2	3	4	5	6	7	8	9	10	11	12	13	14	15	16	17	18	19	20	21	22	23	24	25	26	27	28	29	30	31
JAN																															
FEB																															
MAR																															
APR																															
MAY																															
JUNE																															
JULY																															
AUG																															
SEPT																															
OCT																															
NOV																															
DEC																															

CELBAN WRITING PREPARATION GUIDE

Study Planner

Created by CELBANPrep University
Published by CELBANPrep Publishing

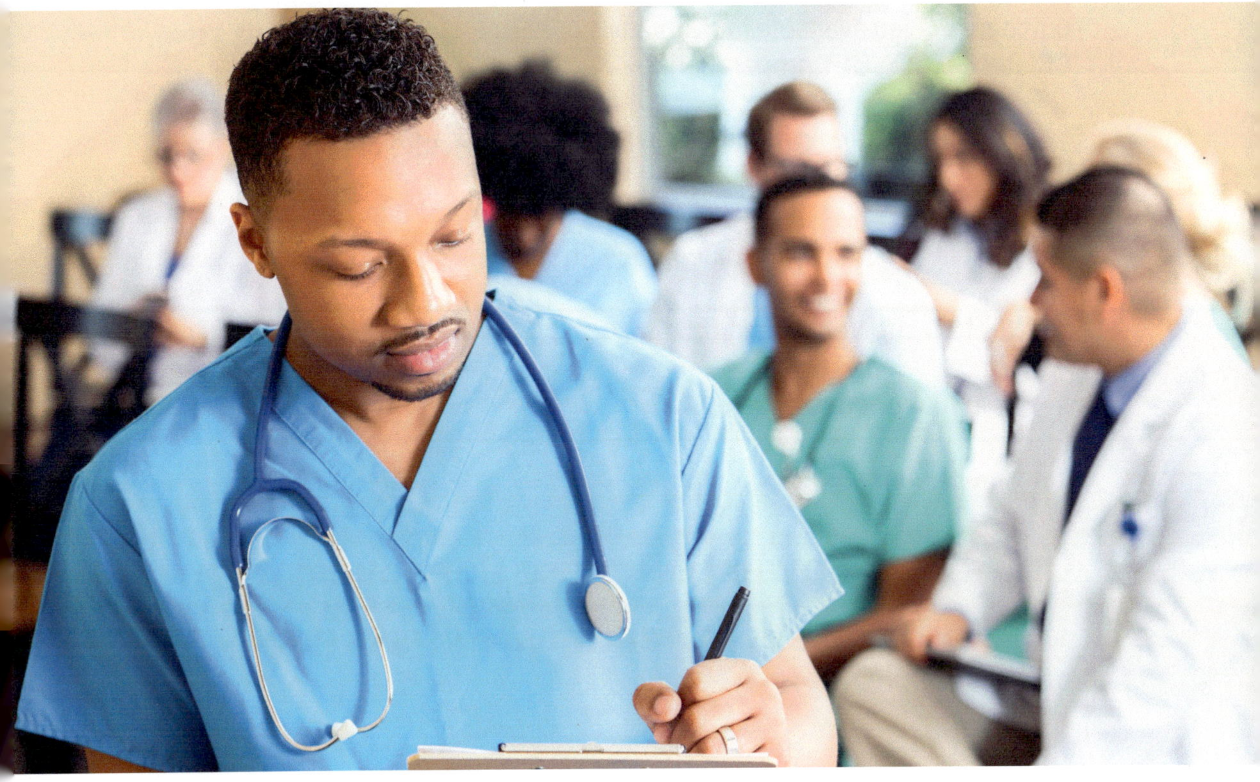

CELBAN WRITING TASK 1 & 2

How to Prepare for the CELBAN

Perfect Medical Grammar

Welcome to CELBANPrep's Medical Grammar

CELBANPrep's Medical Grammar is your indispensable tool for elevating your English language proficiency. In the realm of healthcare, inaccuracies in grammar, punctuation, and sentence structure can result in critical misunderstandings. This comprehensive workbook delves into vital aspects of English grammar.

Enhancing your command over English grammar will empower you to convey ideas with precision, eradicating confusion and enhancing patient outcomes. (Also available individually as CELBAN Grammar Essentials for CELBAN, IELTS, OET preparation.)

To this end, Medical Grammar has been created with Four Modules. They are:

- Perfect Punctuation and Sentence Structure
- Venture into Verbs and Verbals
- Nail Nouns and Articles
- Amplify Agreement

Unlock the Power of Precise Communication: Your success in healthcare starts now!

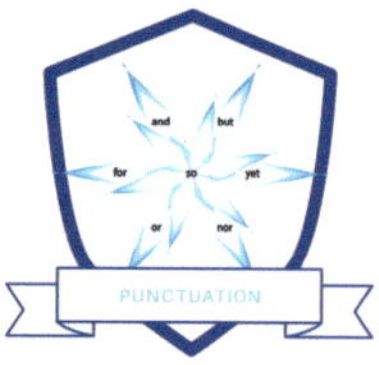

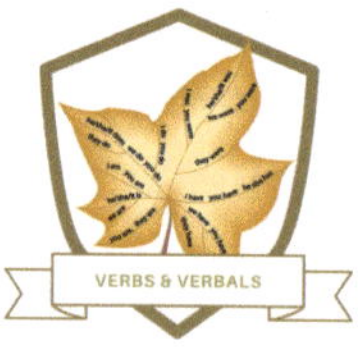

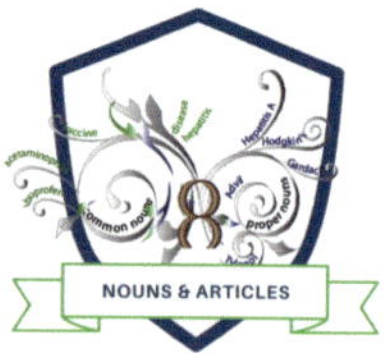

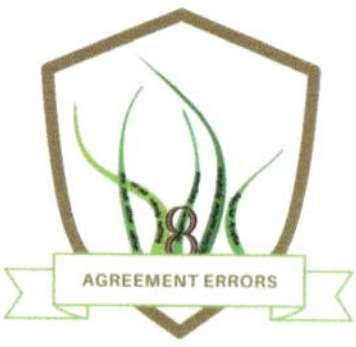

Week One

CELBAN WRITING

INFORMATION

There are several tasks required for the Writing portion of the CELBAN exam. CELBANPrep focuses on a 15-20 minute timed writing task by exploring the Stages of Writing, with an emphasis on learning how to edit your own writing.

CELBANPrep Writing Level One

Writing about Medical Topics

Develop skills in time management, creative writing, and editing.

Improving your writing skills and decreasing your timing are essential to preparing for the written portion of the CELBAN. By applying this four step process, by integrating feedback from a tutor, you will be able to create an organized piece of writing within 15-20 minutes.

CELBANPrep Writing Level Two

Writing in a Medical Context

CELBANPrep Writing Level One is a prerequisites for CELBANPrep Writing Level Two.

Apply the skills you have learned in CELBANPrep Writing Level One to writing in a nursing context: assessments reports, incident reports and completing forms (CELBAN Listening).
It is vital to do the assignment on a daily basis; repetition is key!

It is vital to do the assignment on a daily basis; repetition is key!

CELBAN WRITING

WRITING FLOW CHART

Do you need ways to manage your time and organize your writing?

With four very important stages of writing, how does it relate to the Canadian English Language Benchmark Assessment, the CELBAN?

During the CELBAN you will be given a limited amount of time to complete a writing task. It is important to plan how to use your time to make sure you have time for each of these stages. Here is a rough idea of how CELBANPrep recommends you spend your time.

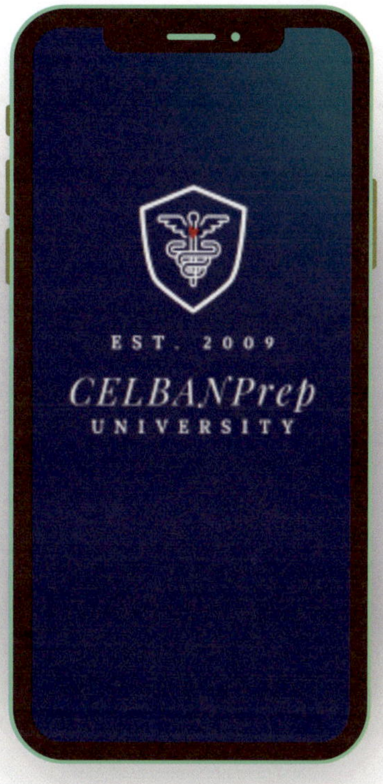

Timing is not everything: practice is essential to be able to write under the CELBAN time constraints. during the exam you are given only 20 minutes! Continue practicing this process until your efficiency increases and you can reach this goal!

Practice is essential to be able to write an organized and detailed report in twenty minutes or less!!!

CELBAN WRITING

WEEK ONE - LESSON ONE

Do you need ways to generate ideas quickly?

Learn how to create an organized and detailed report in less than twenty minutes. Lessons 1-8 of CELBANPrep Writing will teach you how to do this for two tasks:

- writing in a medical context, and
- writing about medical topics.

But first, before we go into that, in Level Two, we need to create and build a strong foundation.

This lesson will teach you how to organize your thoughts within two minutes!

Some people can complete lessons 1-4 in four weeks.
Others take 4 months to learn
how to edit their work: identify their mistakes and correct them.
Take your time.
Be patient.
Whether you realize it or not, you are learning about
patient-centered care from student-centered learning.

CELBAN WRITING

LESSON ONE - PREWRITING

What is the first stage of writing and how can I use it to prepare for CELBAN Writing?

One of the most important steps of writing is pre-writing. Pre-writing is about taking the time to plan what you are going to write about. Without this step, writing is disorganized and missing important elements.

Pre-writing takes practice. The more that you practice the less time it takes to get ideas flowing. When the ideas are flowing it makes it easier to write.

During the writing component of the CELBAN, CELBANPrep recommends that you eventually take 2 minutes for this stage. But, at the beginning you will start by taking 5 minutes to complete this task. This may seem extremely difficult at first. It has been known to take Internationally Educated Nurses up to half an hour to complete a sketch or outline of what they intend to write. CELBANPrep suggests that you practice this stage on a daily basis, for half an hour a day, until you can put together a rough draft of what you will write in two minutes.

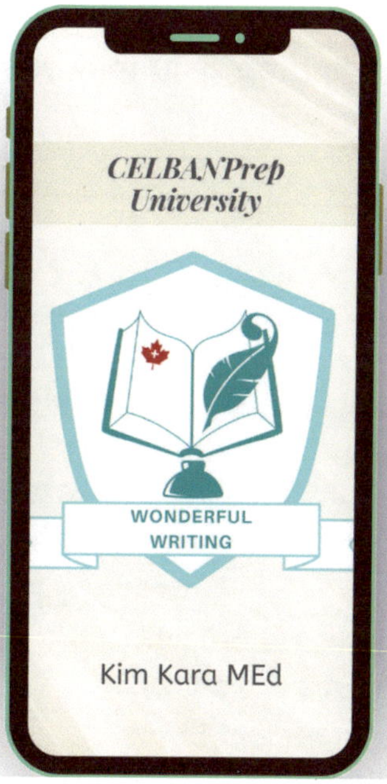

CELBAN WRITING

LESSON ONE - ASSIGNMENT

Do you need to understand how to do this?

So each day you should have 6 mind maps, and 30 by the end of the week.

- 6 maps x 5 minutes = 30 minutes/day
- 6 maps/day x 5 days/week = 30 maps/week

After several weeks you should be able to decrease the amount of time you take to create a Mind Map. **In fact, you will become so good at this process you will be able to do it without paper: in your head!** That is the goal of this lesson.

After two weeks you will be creating Mind Maps in less than two minutes, and then spending 5-10 minutes to write what you have Mind Mapped.

Keep Your Mind Maps!
You will need them for the Second Stage of Writing and the second lesson of CELBANPrep.

Additional resources are available. *CELBAN Grammar Essentials* - available internationally through Amazon - provide tools and resources to assist you in increasing your grammar knowledge when it comes to:

1. Nouns & Articles,
2. Verbs & Verbals,
3. Agreement Errors,
4. Punctuation and Sentence structure.

CELBAN WRITING

LESSON ONE - ASSIGNMENT

Do you need to understand what to do?

For the next week create as many Mind Maps as possible on a variety of topics. Samples, prompts, and starters can be found on the following pages.

- Use the topic ideas you brainstormed earlier. Create at least three mind maps per day; do as many as you can.
- Work until you can create mind maps in 2 minutes or less.
- Continue mind mapping even as you progress to the next lessons. It will make a difference

When you have come to the point where creating a mind map is fast and easy you are ready go to the next stage Lesson Two: Writing.

This mind mapping skill will assist you with CELBAN Speaking as well.

How do I increase my Cohesion Knowledge?

- Begin to increase your cohesion knowledge-base by using mind maps to create organized detailed paragraphs.
- Remember that prewriting is vital; without this step, writing is disorganized and missing important elements.
- Many nurses get low scores on CELBAN Writing because they can not organize their thoughts in the short time given: which wastes time, energy and money.

CELBAN WRITING

BRAINSTORMING RULES

1. Criticism is Ruled Out.
2. *Creative Ideas are Required.*
3. Quality is not Important.
4. *Quantity is Limitless.*
5. Combination is Valued.

CELBAN WRITING

MIND MAPPING EXAMPLES

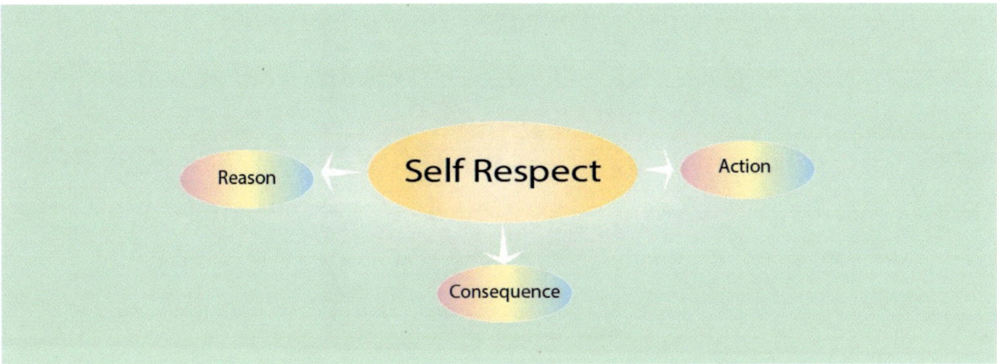

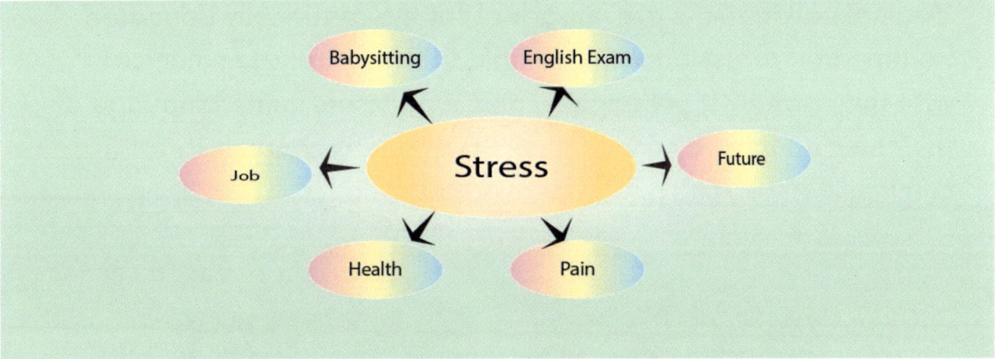

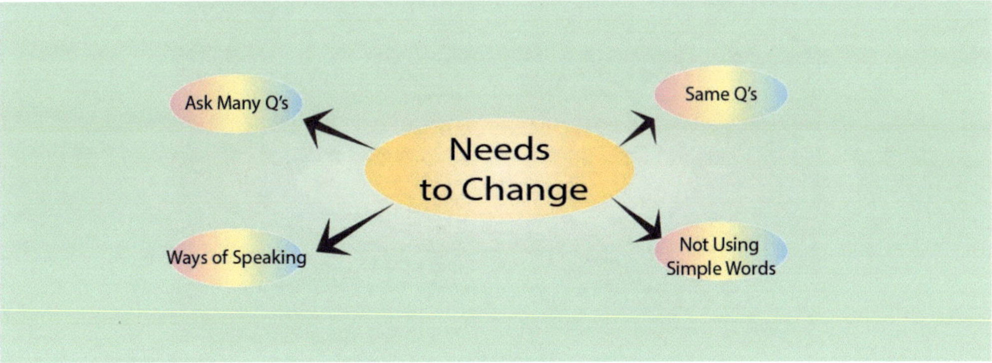

If you run out of ideas,
create a mind map on things you could write about!

MEDICAL COLLOCATION DICTIONARIES

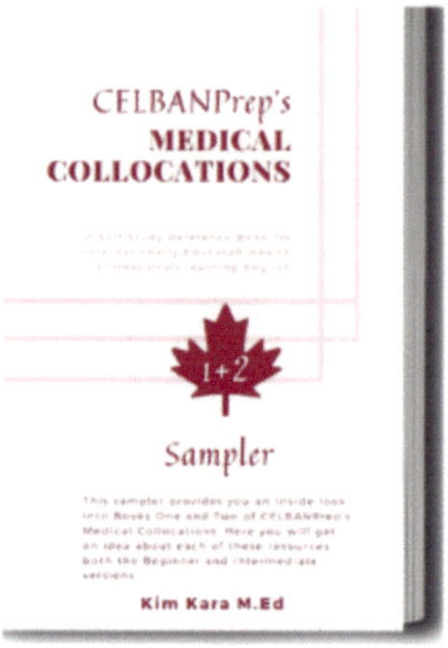

Medical collocations are important for Internationally Educated Healthcare Professionals to be able to effectively communicate with their patients, colleagues, and supervisors in the language of their new country. By using these collocations, you can communicate effectively in the medical field.

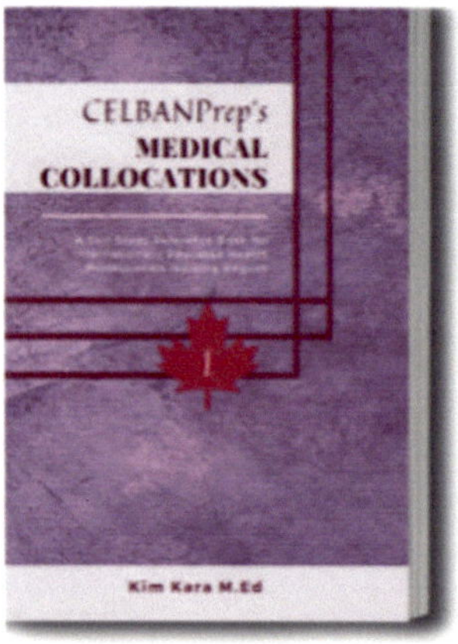

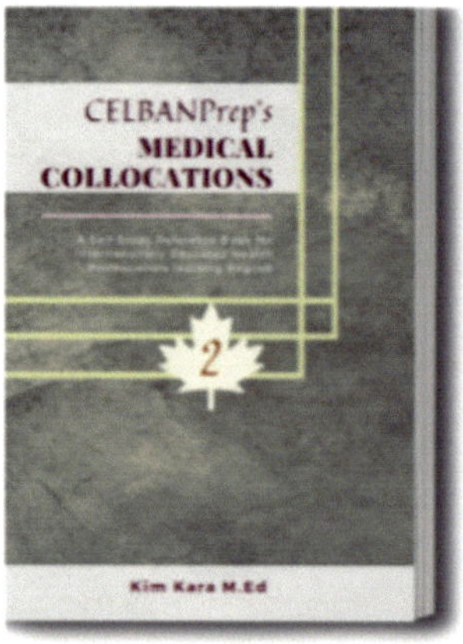

UNLOCK THE POWER OF PRECISE COMMUNICATION:

Your success in healthcare starts now!

Week Two

CELBAN WRITING

WEEK TWO - LESSON TWO

What do I do next?

Now that you have learned how to create a mind map in two minutes, we will go onto the next step: using mindmaps to create organized and detailed pieces of writing.

In this lesson you will see writing that has been created from a mind map. Several examples are presented to you.

It is VITAL to REMEMBER:

- It isn't necessary for you to include all of the ideas you thought about when you created the mindmap.
- The focus is on the writing not editing. Editing is the next stage of writing!
- Learn to choose how much information to take from your mind map, to create a piece of writing. For the CELBAN you need a maximum of two paragraphs. For CELBANPrep you should be able to use your mind map to create one or two brief paragraphs, just like in the examples.
- Remember the goal of this lesson is to write in 5 minutes.
- If you take more 5 minutes you either need more practice, and/or you need to write less.

CELBAN WRITING

WEEK TWO - LESSON TWO

What is the second stage of writing and how can I use it to prepare for CELBAN Writing?

Many people think that Writing is the first and possibly the only stage of writing; this is not true. Writing actually follows Pre-writing, and is strengthened through Editing and cleaned through Rewriting.

During the Writing stage, thoughts and ideas brainstormed during Pre-Writing are brought together. During the CELBAN, CELBANPrep recommends that you spend 5 minutes on this step. Many Internationally Educated Nurses find this difficult at first, but with practice find that it is easy to do.

CELBANPrep reminds you to save time by not worrying about grammar, spelling or sentence structure: these elements can be distracting and interrupt the writing process.

Instead, remember, it is more important to get the ideas down and to correct the spelling, punctuation, sentence structure and add organization during the Editing stage.

Writing is a right brained activity.
Editing is a left brain activity.
Engage one hemisphere of the brain at a time.
You will progress quicker,
and achieve greater success,
when you separate the writing from the editing.

CELBAN WRITING

WEEK TWO - EXAMPLES

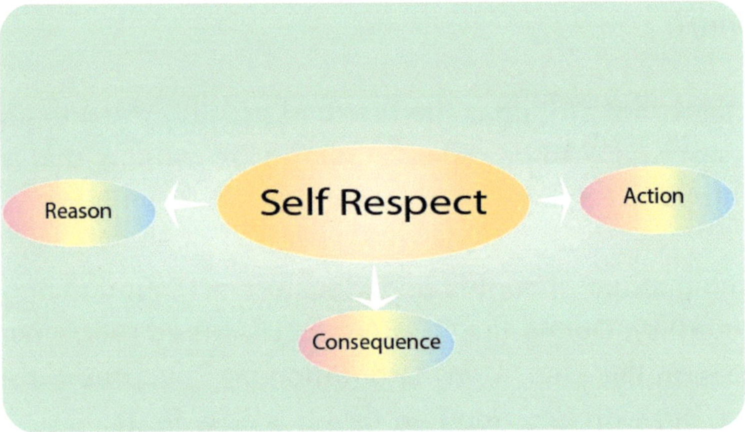

Self Respect

When I came to Canada, to be a nurse is my long time goal. However, English language is my big barrier for me. I was disappointed with my poor English skills. I am hopeless. In order to improve my English skills. I studied LINK program, ESL program and LPN program. After my English studies I have confidence to communicate with different people and learn different experiences from them. I am proud of myself because I step closer to my goal. I need to improve my self respect in being a nurse. Because it can give me confidence to care for my patients and it can help my patients to trust me. In conclusion, improving English skills and nursing knowledge can improve my self respect in Canada.

CELBAN WRITING

WEEK TWO - EXAMPLES

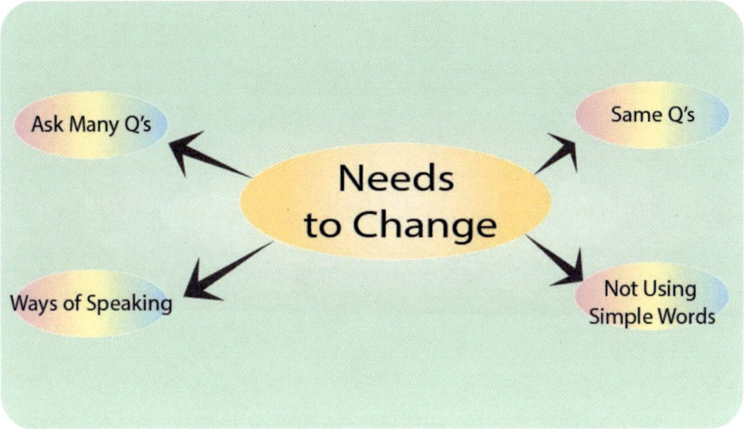

Needs to Change

Being a newcomer to Canada I need to make a change in different times. The most frequent need to be changed is the way of talking or speaking.

Most frequently newcomers mane the same errors in talking or speaking with grammar construction. So to avoid the same error it needs to be changed. Avoiding to ask many questions at the same time, using simple and easy words, and using new words instead of repeated ones are helpful.

If a sentence is constructed grammatically and meaningfully it will be understood easily to everyone and does not need to be repeated. Repetition needs to be changed initially in order to be a good and fluent speaker.

CELBAN WRITING

WEEK TWO - EXAMPLES

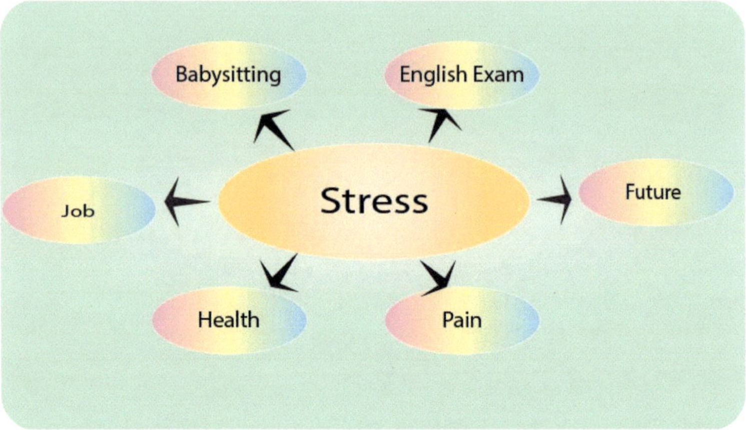

Stress

Stress is part of everybody's life. Today life stress has a very important role in my life. For example baby sitting problems, job, exam, etc. However, I try my best not to think about anything but sometime I end up thinking about it. Consequently my blood pressure in increased. My doctor said I have to watch it. So I decided to change such as listen to music, go for a walk, watch comedy etc. I have to calm down and relax more for my heath and my family.

CELBAN WRITING

WEEK TWO - EXAMPLES

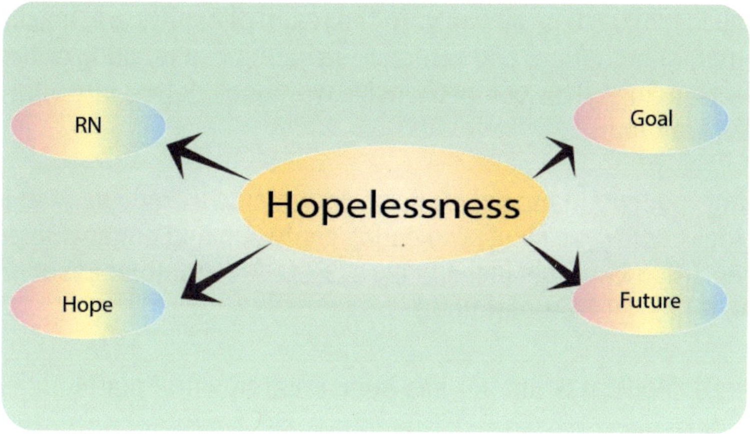

Hopelessness

I was hopeless to gain a lifelong career so I decided to upgrade my nursing degree here in Canada. For a while I have a job in a restaurant but I find it difficult because the workers just come and go. The manager and the boss did not come to work every time. We were short of staff and it is very hard to have new workers all the time. I have decided to stay with CELBANPrep because we have the same goal in our life and strive for hope in the future.

Perfect Medical Grammar

Welcome to CELBANPrep's Medical Grammar

CELBANPrep's Medical Grammar is your indispensable tool for elevating your English language proficiency. In the realm of healthcare, inaccuracies in grammar, punctuation, and sentence structure can result in critical misunderstandings. This comprehensive workbook delves into vital aspects of English grammar.

Enhancing your command over English grammar will empower you to convey ideas with precision, eradicating confusion and enhancing patient outcomes. (Also available individually as CELBAN Grammar Essentials for CELBAN, IELTS, OET preparation.)

To this end, Medical Grammar has been created with Four Modules. They are:

- Perfect Punctuation and Sentence Structure
- Venture into Verbs and Verbals
- Nail Nouns and Articles
- Amplify Agreement

Unlock the Power of Precise Communication: Your success in healthcare starts now!

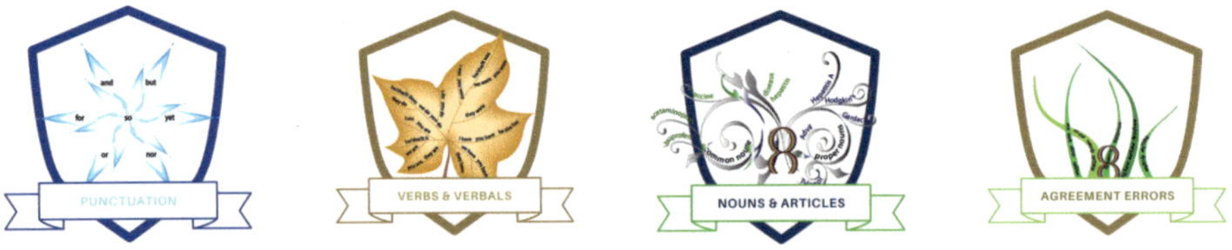

One of the things

YOU ARE BEING ASSESSED ON

during the CELBAN

IS YOUR ABILITY TO

follow

instructions.

CELBANPrep

IS

no different.

You

MUST

follow instructions.

CELBAN WRITING

WEEK TWO - ASSIGNMENT

How do I practice Writing About Medical Topics?

- Set your timer for 5 minutes.
- Using a mind map you created in the Pre-Writing Stage, prepare to write a paragraph.
- Looking at the mind map decide which topics you have enough details to write about.
- Choose one of the topics and begin to write.
- **Do not stop or worry about grammar, punctuation or spelling.**
- Write until you have nothing else to add.
- Ensure that you spend half an hour a day using mindmaps to create writing: 30 minutes divided by 5 minutes per topic = 6 topics.

REMEMBER:

- It isn't necessary for you to include all of the ideas you thought about when you created the mindmap.
- Also, the focus is on the writing not editing. ***Editing is the next stage of writing!***
- Learn to choose how much information to take from your mind map, to create a piece of writing. For the CELBAN you need a maximum of two paragraphs. For CELBANPrep you should be able to use your mind map to create one or two brief paragraphs, just like in the examples.
- Remember the goal of this lesson is to write in 5 minutes.
- If you take more 5 minutes you either need more practice, and/or you need to write less.

Week Three

CELBAN WRITING

WEEK THREE- LESSON THREE

How do I increase my score in writing?

By now you have completed two of the fundamental stages of writing. Your brain is working faster at creating mind maps and turning them into writing. During the last stage, you were asked to write without worrying about grammar, punctuation, or organization. This is part of the third stage: editing.

Remember how a score of 5-8 on the CELBAN/CLB means that you have intermediate skills, and can communicate in a moderately demanding situation? Self-correcting (whether in writing or when speaking) is an advanced skill that many beginners can not do, and advanced communicators do unconsciously competently: without thinking.

Thus, learn how to edit your written work.
Editing is an advanced skill. It is a perfect way to demonstrate that you are, indeed, at an intermediate level of writing in the English language.

For this lesson, you will be reviewing your work looking for errors and correcting them.

At first it may take you longer than 5 minutes to edit,
but by using the CELBANPrep *Grammar Essentials*,
and applying the stages of writing to medical topics,
for 30 minutes a day,
in time it will take you less time to edit your work.

CELBAN WRITING

WEEK THREE - INTEGRATING FEEDBACK

How do I learn how to correct my mistakes?

One of the things that makes the CELBAN different from any other English exam is that it was created in Canada, for Internationally Educated Nurses, that seek to be licensed in Canada. That is what the "C" in CELBAN stands for: Canada/Canadian.

As such, the CELBAN has been infused with the values of the Canadian education system: where we apply learner-centred practices to assist our students in improving their skills. For that reason, when you sit for the CELBAN along with your score you will get a report that includes feedback on what you need to improve. Some of the comments, about your writing and speaking skills may be: problems with sentence structure, incorrect sentence structure, article errors, inconsistent verb tense, and/or agreement errors.

CELBANPrep's *Grammar Essentials* series was created to assist you in learning how to edit your work, and stop making those kinds of mistakes. There is one module, one volume, for each of the following common weaknesses of Internationally Educated Nurses:

- Nouns & Articles, Verbs & Verbals,
- Agreement Errors,
- Punctuation & Sentence Structure.

If you have not already used these modules, start now.

CELBAN WRITING

WEEK THREE - ASSIGNMENT

What is the third stage of writing and how can I use it to prepare for CELBAN Writing?

Editing is the step that follows Writing. It is one of the most important stages and should not be forgotten. It is fundamental to give yourself time to edit your work: this is key to improving your results.

For this assignment, you will be taking pieces of writing you have already written, and editing them for grammar, punctuation, and organization.

At this stage, the number of errors you have should be decreasing as you integrate what you have learned about your personal weaknesses. By using the CELBANPrep's *Grammar Essentials* module that addresses where you as an individual need to improve: you will not only be able to identify your mistakes but also know how to correct them. The triaging process will help you to figure out how to:

- use complex sentence structures, with only a few errors.
- capitalize correctly.
- use phrases and connectors correctly.
- use phrases and connectors correctly.
- keep your verb tense consistent.
- avoid making agreement errors.

CELBAN WRITING

WEEK THREE - SELF EVALUATION

How do I evaluate my own writing?

To be able to edit your own work, you need to be able to identify your own common mistakes:

- Have you used punctuation correctly?
- Have you kept the verb tenses consistent: either all in the present or all in the past?
- If you do not know how to spell a word, can you think of other words that mean the same thing?
- Are the sentences and paragraphs organized in a way that makes sense and allows a fluid read?
- Have you followed the appropriate format?

Having a second set of skilled and encouraging eyes may be helpful.

Two of the most important test-taking strategies to pass CELBAN writing are:
1. time management to allow time for
2. editing.

You can increase your score tremendously by finding and correcting your errors.

If you have not already done so ensure that you get a copy of CELBANPrep's *Grammar Essentials* as companion resources to CELBANPrep.

CELBAN WRITING

WEEK THREE - EXAMPLES

Can I see examples of an IEN using this editing stage of writing?

Life in Canada

In Canada there was four seasons, they are winter, spring, summer and fall. In the winter it is especially cold. People have been to wear a coat,s boots, hats, some mittens, and a scarf. There are some activitie you can do in winter in Canada that we do not do back home. There is skiing, skating, making snow forts, making snow angels, and have snow ball fights, wnd making snowmen.

There are a couple of things that need to be corrected. Here is the edited version. Look for the changes:

In Canada there are four seasons: they are winter, spring, summer and fall. In the winter it is especially cold. People have to wear a coat, boots, hats, some mittens, and a scarf. There are some activities you can do in the winter in Canada that we do not do back home. Adults often go skiing and skating. Children can be found making snow forts, snow angels, snowmen or having snow ball fights.

It also needs a conclusion:

Although winters in Canada are cold, people can dress warm and have fun.

CELBAN WRITING

WEEK THREE - TIPS & TRICKS

How do I edit my own writing?

During the editing stage, you will focus on bringing clarity and organization to what you wrote. It is important to check each of the following elements one at a time:

- spelling/typing,
- capitalization
- grammar,
- punctuation, and
- organization.

But, at the beginning, it may be too difficult for you to search for all of them at the same time. Our brains do not work like that. First, we have to create a search image: an image of what we are searching for. Let's say, for example, our search image is for articles. Thus, when we read what we wrote, we skim we look for articles. When we find one, we stop and analyze it knowing what we learned from the triaging process in the CELBANPrep *Grammar Essentials* series. We leave it if it is correct or change it if appropriate. Then we look for the next article. We repeat the process. When this is done we go on to assess our next weakness. In this way we create separate search images for each error we make until eventually the synapses in our brain are so strong that we self-correct without thinking about it, then we stop making the mistake altogether.

CELBAN WRITING

WEEK THREE - MORE TIPS FOR SUCCESS

When can I move on to CELBANPrep Writing Level Two: writing in a nursing context?

- Use the "A Year in Pixels" to track when you spend at least 30 minutes a day doing editing work that you created for the previous lesson.
- Spend a maximum of 10 minutes editing per piece. If it takes longer start writing shorter pieces. (The longer the piece the more corrections you have to make. Start short. Then when you are quicker at editing, and writing, you can start adding a few sentences at a time.)
- Ensure that you integrate the feedback you have received on your writing. Spend some time making edits and resubmitting the assignments to a qualified tutor.
- Use CELBANPrep's *Grammar Essentials* to turn your weaknesses into strengths.

Do not advance to CELBANPrep Writing Level Two until you can identify your own errors and correct them. When you have achieved mastery, you are ready to advance to the next stage.

To continue on to Writing Level Two (lessons 5-8) you must be able to:

- correct your own work,
- have very few errors in grammar, spelling and punctuation.
- make only minor errors when it comes to collocations is acceptable.

Week Four

CELBAN WRITING

WEEK FOUR - LESSON FOUR

How do I organize my writing?

During the last lesson you learned:

- it is important that you have the skills and abilities to improve your writing. To do so you have to be aware of the grammar and punctuation rules.
- to take time to review what you wrote in the Writing Stage. Edit for spelling, grammar and punctuation.
- to edit your work, daily, until you can do so within 5 minutes.

But what we did not cover is organization techniques:

- Inserting an introductory sentence and a concluding one, if you had not already done so.

By now your writing has a sense of organization simply because of the mindmapping that you did during lesson one, week one. By creating mind maps of your thoughts, ideas, feelings and opinions about medical topics, before you write, you intrinsically create an internal organizational system. But, there is one more step to polish off your piece of writing: adding a solid introduction and conclusion.

Start with familiar topics, that are easy to think about and write about. Then, when you are ready, start writing about medical topics.

CELBAN WRITING

WEEK FOUR - LESSON FOUR

Do I write the introduction at the beginning or after I finish writing the piece?

What you may have realized is that what you have been learning about the stages of writing is that writing is a creative process that requires both the left and the right brain.

- The left hemisphere is logical, convergent, and sequential.
- The right hemisphere is creative, divergent, and holistic.

Mind mapping is right-brained.
Writing is right-brained.
Editing is left-brained.

But what about writing the introduction and the conclusion?

Many left-brained people - both students and teachers - start writing with an outline. So they write the introduction before they start writing and add the conclusion at the end. Right-brained learners and creatives create the introduction at the end, at the same time as the conclusion, because the reality is that they do not know what they are going to write until it is written.

If writing an introduction and conclusion is difficult for you, then experiment with writing the introduction and conclusion *after* you have written the content.

CELBAN WRITING

WEEK FOUR - ORGANIZATION

What is the best way to add organization to a piece of writing?

The answer to that question comes back to lesson #1 on mindmapping.

1. *The Main Topic*

   When you mind map, you put the main topic in the center: that word or phrase goes in the title, the introduction and the conclusion of the piece you are writing.

2. *Topic Sentences*

   The next thing you do, when mind mapping, is create the subtopics. The subtopics then transform into topic sentences.

3. *Body Content*

   The rest of the information in the mind map goes into the body of the text. It becomes the main content.

Ultimately, by creating mind maps, you already have a structure.

Would you like to see an example?

CELBAN WRITING

WEEK FOUR - EXAMPLE

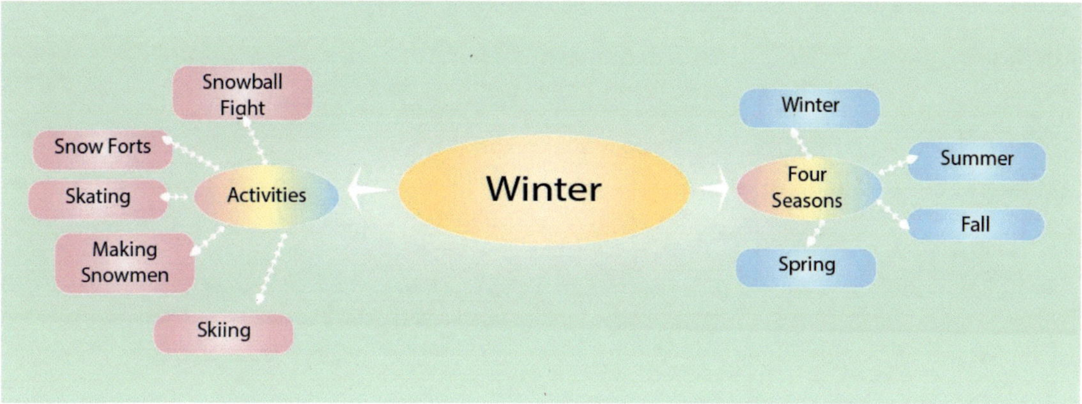

Skill Practice: Winter

Use this mind map about winters in Canada to determine:

- a title based on the topic (in the centre),
- the topic sentences for the two paragraphs (the rainbow ovals),
- the details to be expanded on:
    - paragraph A (in pink), and
    - paragraph B (in blue).

Use the stages of writing, time yourself, write about Canadian winters.

Then, use this information to write the introduction and the conclusion.

When you are done, read the short piece on the following page. It will be very different from what you wrote. Still, you will be able to identify the parts and imagine the possibilities.

CELBAN WRITING

WEEK FOUR - WRITTEN EXAMPLE

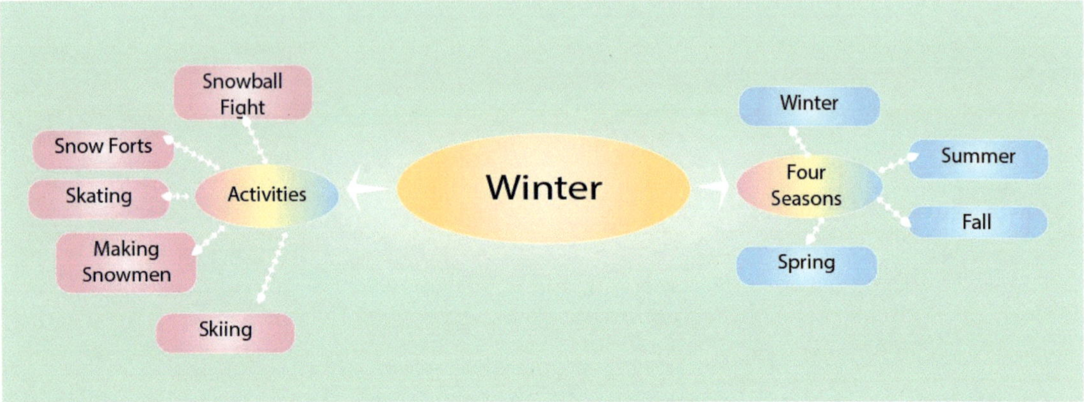

Winter

Life in Canada is different from living in other areas of the world. One thing that stands out about Canada is the winter season. There are two things to explore. One is the duration of this season. The other is activities we can do during the winter season.

One of the things about life in Canada is that there are four seasons: winter, spring, summer, and fall. But, the length and duration of each season depends on where in Canada one lives. In some places, each season is 3 months long. In other parts of Canada winter can last 8 months or even longer.

Yet, there are many activities that make long winters more enjoyable. With snow we can make snowmen, forts, and have snow ball fights. Skating and skiing are other activities, even sports, that can be enjoyed with friends and family.

So, when people move to Canada, it is important to consider the location and the duration of the winter season because engaging in winter sports can be lots of fun.

Winter

CELBAN WRITING

WEEK FOUR - ASSIGNMENT

How do I apply this to my own writing?

There are two things you can do:

1. review the pieces you have already written, or
2. write another piece from the start.

A. Review the Pieces you have Already Written

Analyze what you have written.

- Ensure the title is based on the main topic.
- Check to see if you wrote topic sentences. Are they based on the subtopics in the mind map? Rewrite it/them as necessary.
- Have you written an introduction and conclusion? Use the structure of the mindmap to write or rewrite them as necessary.

B. Write Another Piece from the start.

- **2 min:** create a mind map
- **5 min:** write a title based on the topic (in the centre)
    - draft a topic sentence from the subheadings,
    - use the details to write the body of the paragraph,
    - add a suitable introduction and conclusion.
- **5 min:** edit your work.

CELBAN WRITING PREPARATION GUIDE

Congratulations

Created by CELBANPrep University
Published by CELBANPrep Publishing

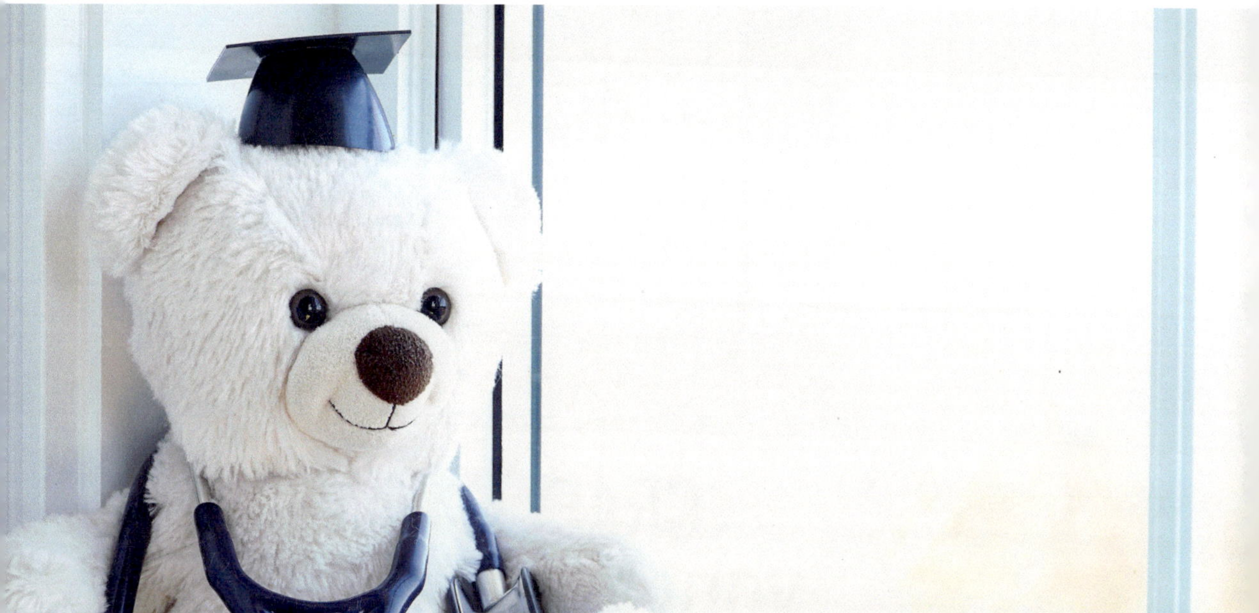

YOU HAVE COMPLETED CELBANPREP WRITING LEVEL ONE

On to CELBANPrep Writing Level Two

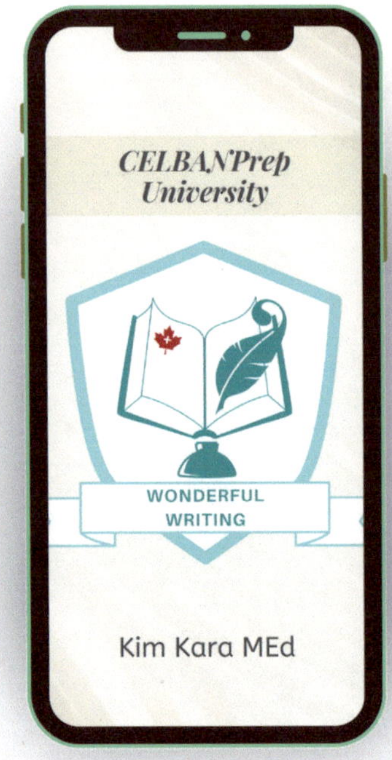

CRAFT YOUR WORDS

MASTER THE ART OF WONDERFUL WRITING

CELBAN WRITING PREPARATION GUIDE

Study Planner

Created by CELBANPrep University
Published by CELBANPrep Publishing

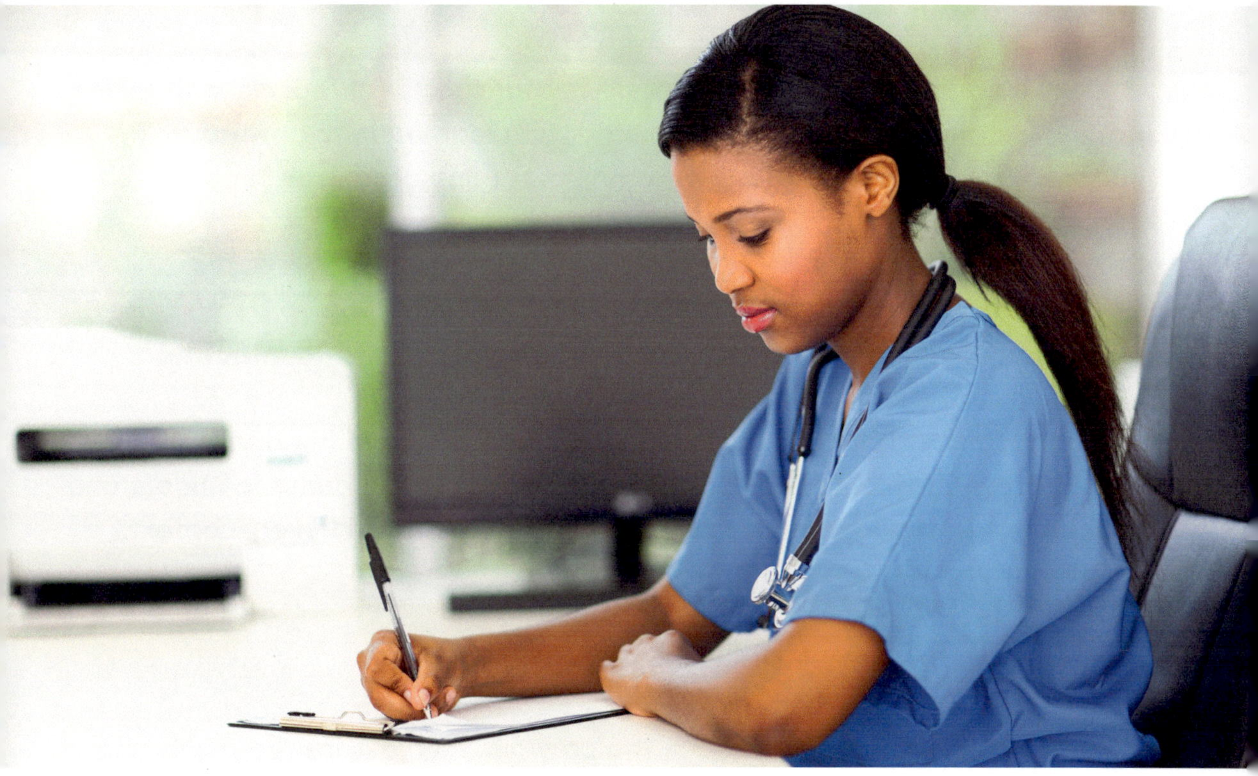

CELBAN WRITING LEVEL TWO (MEDICAL REPORTS)

How to Prepare for the CELBAN

CELBAN WRITING

INTRODUCTION - WRITING LEVEL TWO

How do I apply everything I have learned to writing in a nursing context?

Earlier in this book, you were prompted to "Create a list of incidents and brief patient descriptions that you can write about as a medical report." Now you will have the opportunity to apply the stages of writing to a medical context.

This will be done through two different formats: incident reports, and taking patient histories. When you apply the skill you learned in the previous chapters, you will be able to write a complete and organized report in 20 minutes or less.

The ultimate goal of CELBANPrep Writing is for you to be able to complete a detailed and organized report in 12-15 minutes.

To do this, instead of mind mapping what you will be writing about, you will be given two different flow charts. By doing so, you will come to understand how easy it is to adapt what you have learned to any and every context:

- at home, at work, and in the community;
- when you are writing and when you are speaking.

Thus, the skills you have learned in the previous four lessons are highly transferable. They are the foundation of any clear communicator. They are the foundation of any successful career and life.

CELBAN WRITING

INTRODUCTION - CELBANPREP WRITING

What is CELBANPrep Writing Level Two about? How is it different from Level One?

When you become a registered nurse in Canada, there are many steps to your process. Providing the required Language Efficiency score is only the beginning. Even after such time, you may be required to take courses, workshops, do clinicals, and the like.

In order to function in Canadian medical services, you must have skills and abilities that are consistent with our culture. The CELBAN is one step in that direction of acquiring the communication skills that increase your competency when connecting with other medical professionals, members of the community, patients, and the like.

In this way, the CELBAN can be considered a way to ease your entry into your career.

It can not be considered equivalent to the IELTS because the IELTS does not have that career aspect. It is not about easing your process into life as a medical professional in Canada. And it does not address the needs of patients and hospitals in Canada. In fact, errors in communication in the medical field can be fatal. Acting inconsistent with the Canadian culture can lead to legal proceedings. That is why the scores you are required to obtain, on the CELBAN, are so high.

CELBAN WRITING

INTRODUCTION - SCORES

Why are the scores on the CELBAN so high?

It is important to understand the answer to this question so that you fully value the CELBAN as a career entry channel.

Taking time to increase your competencies in reading, writing, listening and speaking will take you father in your career (whatever it may be).
The CELBAN acts as a safeguard to patients, hospitals, and other medical professionals.
It is vital to spend ample time studying, preparing, practicing, overcoming and achieving.
To do so not only increases your competencies, it increases your confidence to communicate with staff, patients and their families: in English.

When you become a licensed nurse, in Canada, you will be grateful for these skills that will allow you to communicate - in writing and speaking - with greater competence and confidence.

CELBAN WRITING

INTRODUCTION - REVIEW

What do I need to know?

During the CELBAN you have time to write a report.

CELBANPrep Writing Level One teaches you the time management, creative writing, and editing skills required to be able to complete a well written, organized report in the allotted amount of time: spending some of that time editing your work, identifying and correcting errors in grammar, punctuation and capitalization.

You have already brainstormed not only a list of topics you can write incident reports about, but you have also brainstormed a list of sources where you can get more ideas.

So, before we go into the stages of writing in a nursing context, let us review the skills and competencies that the CELBAN/CLB has been created to assess. Remember: some skills are required in all tasks, other skills are specific to a task.

When it comes to writing a medical report you are demonstrating your knowledge when it comes to grammar, cohesion and interpreting inference. You are also given an opportunity to demonstrate your social and emotional intelligence while interacting with others and giving/understanding instructions. The list of skills follow on the next two pages.

All TASKS:

- **Grammar Knowledge**
- **Cohesion Knowledge**
- **Interpretive Knowledge**
- **Emotional Intelligence**
- **Social Intelligence**

Skills to be demonstrated:

Create a coherent piece of writing.

Communicate, in writing, with an appropriate tone and language.

Communicate both implicit and explicit meanings, in writing.

Express main ideas with supporting details, examples, or stories.

Use complex stentence structures, with only a few errors.

Use phrases and connectors correctly.

Spell and capitalize correctly.

Use punctuation correctly.

Use articles correctly.

Keep your verb tense consistent.

Avoid making agreement errors.

Writing a Medical Report

- Interacting with Others
- Giving/Understanding Instructions

Skills to be demonstrated:

Write in a way that communicates what you understand.

Write clearly and accurately in a moderately demanding situation.

Communicate, in writing, with an appropriate tone and language.

Communicate clear direction and instructions.

Explain a sequence of events clearly and accurately.

Express main ideas with supporting details.

Use appropriate sentence structure, with only a few errors.

Write numbers correctly.

Use abbreviations correctly.

Use medical phrases correctly.

Skill Practice

Traditionally the assessment of an IENs ability to interact with others, and understand instructions happens through a medical report. We will explore incident reports and assessment reports.

CELBAN WRITING

INTRODUCTION - WRITING IN A MEDICAL CONTEXT

How do I apply the writing stage to a nursing context?

The stages of writing are the same, regardless of the topic. Previously CELBANPrep has focused on applying the stages of writing to topics about medical topics with the understanding that it is extremely difficult for many Internationally Educated Nurses to write creatively.

Writing, for professionals in the medical field, is not about ***creating*** facts, situations, and scenarios. To medical professionals writing is about ***reporting*** facts, observations, and actions.

That is why CELBANPrep Writing Level One acknowledges that it takes time and practice to write creatively. Where the written component of the CELBAN is nursing-related, it takes a degree of creative thinking to be able to complete the tasks required of this portion of the English Language assessment.

There are two different types of reports you will be taught to write through CELBANPrep Writing Level Two: Intake Assessment and Incident Report. In this way, you will learn a transferable skill that will allow you to excel on the exam regardless of the question they ask you. You will have and maintain confidence without experiencing additional stress or tension during the exam.

Week Five

One of the things

YOU ARE BEING ASSESSED ON,

during the CELBAN,

IS YOUR ABILITY TO

follow

instructions.

CELBANPrep

IS

no different.

You

MUST

follow instructions.

CELBAN WRITING

WEEK FIVE - MAPPING A REPORT

How can I use the prewriting stage in a nursing context?

Prewriting creates organization in writing.
Mind Maps can be used to organize writing in a nursing context.

What do you include in an incident report?

Typically you would include the following information:

- Observations,
- Your Assessment,
- Medical Interventions, and
- Documentation.

We will go through one aspect at a time, developing mind maps as we go.

IENs that do not apply the stages of writing
end up writing
incomplete reports,
run out of time, or
hand in the report filled with errors.

CELBAN WRITING

WEEK FIVE - OBSERVATIONS

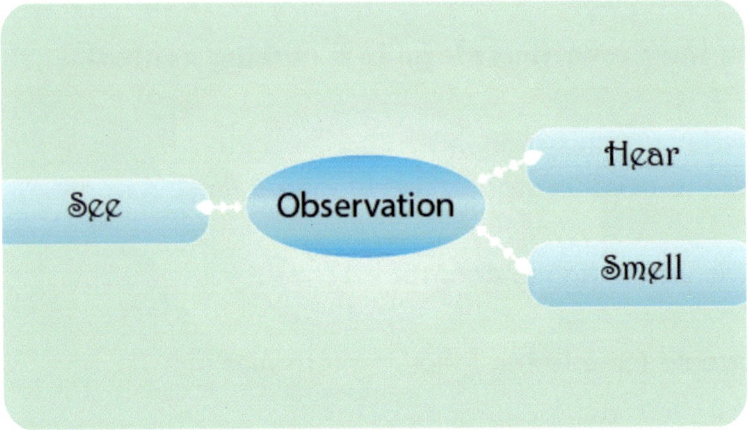

Observations

Observations are an important part of an incident report. Observations include what you see, hear and smell when you arrive on the scene. This can be mind mapped.

Without CELBANPrep many IENs forget to add these details in their report. Others create assumptions in what they write.

When seeing an elderly patient on the floor an IEN might write that the patient fell, but this is an assumption. There are many explanations for why the patient is on the floor: being pushed, looking for something, or something else. Unless a witness said, "The patient fell," it has to be worded differently. You can either write that the patient told you he fell, or that a witness told you, or that you simply found him on the floor.

CELBAN WRITING

WEEK FIVE - ASSESSMENT

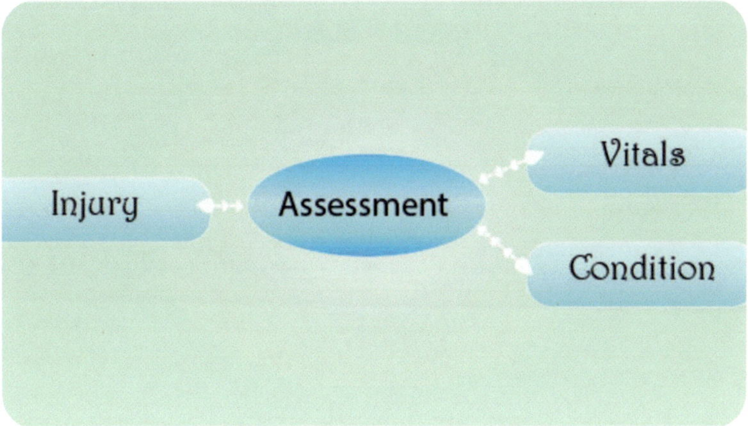

Assessment

As a nurse, what is the next thing you do when you arrive at the scene of an incident at work? First, observe the situation, then assess the patient.

What are some of the things you do during an assessment?

- Check vitals.
- Check condition.
- Look for injuries.

Create a mind map using these aspects. If you were to add to this mind map, from vitals you could simply draw lines branching out, and write blood pressure, temperature, respiratory rate, and pulse. You can also add the actual rates.

CELBAN WRITING

WEEK FIVE - INTERVENTION

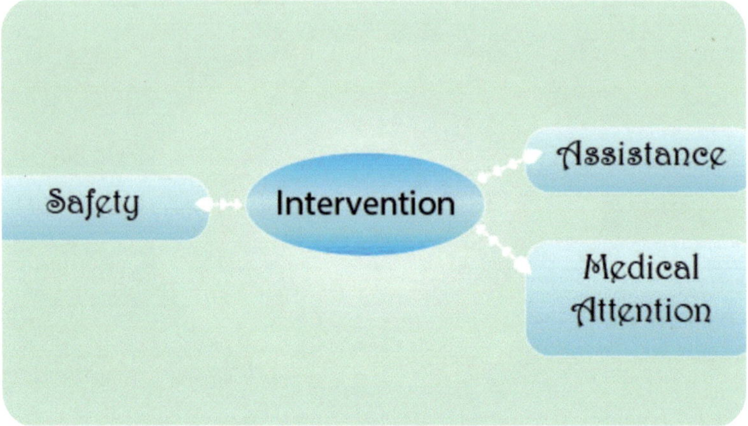

Intervention

Once the patient has been assessed, as an RN, you would provide medical interventions. This would include: ensuring safety, calling for assistance, and providing medical attention. You can also include the outcome of the intervention, such as stabilized vitals. In this section, you would note informing the doctor, the doctor's orders, medication given (name and dose).

CELBAN WRITING

WEEK FIVE - DOCUMENTATION

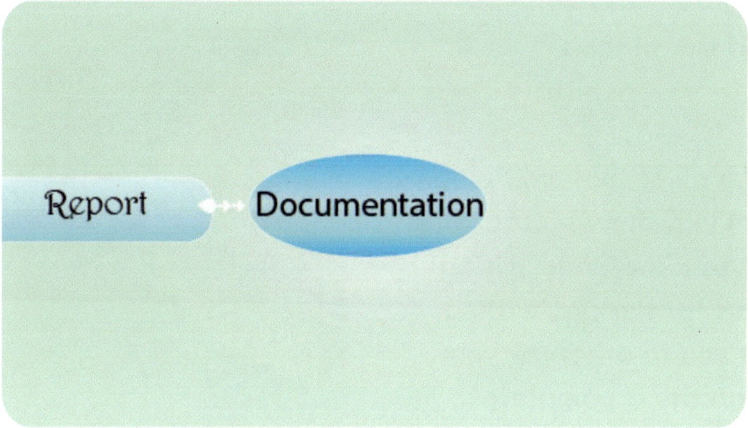

Documentation

Without CELBANPrep most IENs do not add documentation in their incident report. Yet this is an important nursing standard. Appropriate documentation is vital for complete reports and continuity in care. A simple mind map is as follows:

Examples include:

- beginning a blood sugar chart,
- charting continuous monitoring,
- hourly observations, and
- input/output.

What other kinds of reports or charts would you use.

CELBAN WRITING

WEEK FIVE - FLOW CHART

How do I put the pieces together?

When we take all of the mind maps and link them in order we create an Incident Report Flow Chart. Using this flow chart for the pre-writing stage allows you to organize your thoughts to create a complete report that is consistent with documentation standards. Using this flow chart for the pre-writing stage allows you to organize your thoughts.

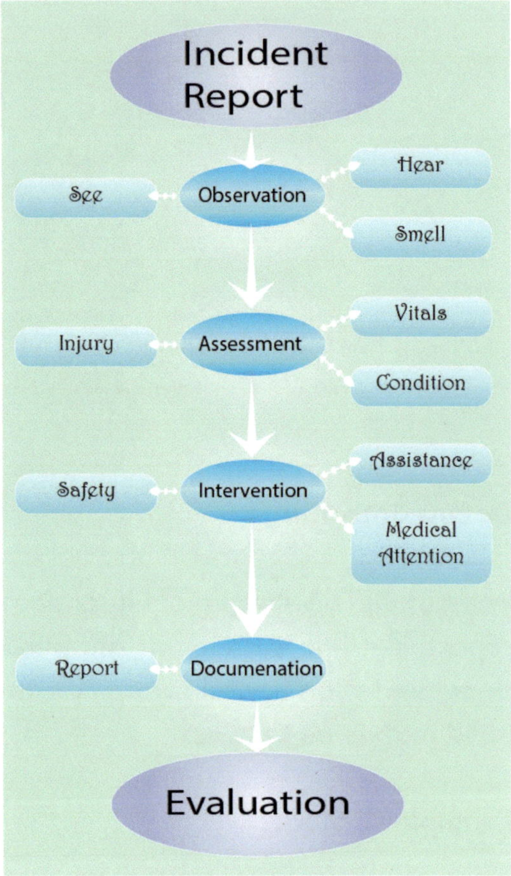

CELBAN WRITING

WEEK FIVE - ABOUT THE ASSIGNMENT

How do I do this: write an incident report?

Your assignment is to continue applying the stages of writing, using the Incident Report Flow Chart to organize your thoughts and ideas. You will be required to time yourself, making sure you have time to edit your work.

IENs that do not apply the stages of writing end up:

- writing incomplete reports,
- running out of time,
- or handing in a report filled with errors.

Applying the stages of writing to writing incident reports allows you to:

- write complete reports with details.
- use time effectively.
- correct errors before handing in the exam.

At first, you will simply create incident report flow charts, similar to how in week one all you did was mind mapping. Each day you will create 6 flow charts, a total of 30 by the end of the week.

- 6 maps x 5 minutes = 30 minutes/day
- 6 maps/day x 5 days/week = 30 maps/week

CELBAN WRITING

WEEK FIVE - ASSIGNMENT

How do I start my report?

Using flow charts for prewriting in a nursing context creates organization and ensures that the incident report you write is complete and detailed.

On a daily basis spend at least half an hour a day adding details to the flow charts to create incident reports that you can write about. Allow a maximum of 5 minutes per flow chart.

Here are some writing prompts:

- A 65-year-old man: found on the floor by the elevator with an IV pole.
- 6-year-old girl: found on the floor in the bathroom, a wet pool of liquid is on the floor.
- A 16-year-old: found on the ground near the hand sanitizing station.
- Create your own incident(s) based on experience, observation, or a scene from a movie or television show.

Complete as many flow charts as required until you can complete one in two minutes or less.

On a daily basis
spend at least half an hour a day
creating flow charts for incident reports that you can write
about for the following lesson.

Week Six

CELBAN WRITING

WEEK SIX - WRITING A REPORT

When can I start writing incident reports?

Continue with the assignment for week five until you can complete one in two minutes or less.

- You may be able to do this in one week.
- It may take you a matter of several weeks.

Either way, start converting your flowcharts into actual incident reports when you are able to generate your flow chart both quickly and easily.

It is even better if you can map out your thoughts and ideas in your head (without using paper or a computer.)

This is a highly advanced skill, that will assist you tremendously in achieving your goals in life.

INSTRUCTIONS:

Once you are able to create your incident report charts quickly, apply the following stage of writing.

- Set the timer for 5 minutes.
- Using one of the flow charts you created, write for 5 minutes.
- Stop.
- Edit your writing for the final 5 minutes.

CELBAN WRITING

WEEK SIX - HOW

How do I transform a flow chart into a report?

What you will realize is that what you have been taught through CELBANPrep Writing Level One is that you are able to accomplish a great deal in a short amount of time.

If it takes 15 minutes to write a report, each day you will write 2 reports. By the end of the week, you will have completed and edited 10 reports.

- 2 reports x 15 minutes = 30 minutes/day
- 2 reports/day x 5 days/week = 10 reports/week

After several weeks you should be able to decrease the amount of time you take to create the flow charts and write the reports. In time your reports will be longer because of how competent you get with these skills.

CELBAN WRITING

WEEK SIX - EDITING A MEDICAL REPORT

How do I apply the other stages of writing?

Now that you have used the Incident Flow Chart to organize your thoughts for the prewriting lesson, you will apply the other stages of writing to learn how to write in a time-efficient manner.

Make sure you take the time to edit your report: spot errors and correct them to increase your score. You must be able to self-correct grammar, spelling, punctuation, and capitals for this lesson.

The last lesson of CELBANPrep Writing introduced the skill of using a mind map to organize your thoughts and ideas in relation to writing an incident report. Here you followed a step-by-step process of creating individual mind maps towards linking them together in an Incident Report Flow Chart.

Having understood the usefulness of this skill, using mind mapping for brainstorming in previous weeks, you will soon find comfort and ease in writing a complete incident report in less than twenty minutes: including time for editing and revising.

See examples of incident reports written by Internationally Educated Nurses on the following pages. You can also read the debriefing about the errors that were written within the report.

Learn some evaluation criteria, and then take a turn identifying errors.

CELBAN WRITING

WEEK SIX - EXAMPLE - KNOW YOUR ROLE

Incident: A 16 year old found on the ground near the hand sanitizing station.

On May 19, at 8:00 am, a male teenager was found on the ground screaming for help. Palelooking, crying in pain. A few minutes later found to be gasping for breath. Radial pulse taken, 50 bpm. Ambulance was called. After 15 minutesthe ambulance came, took vital signs, BP taken 120/60, P-60 bpm. Sent to the hospital for further assessment. ---------------------- signature

Debriefing

This IEN was fortunate to take CELBANPrep before her exam. She did not understand the instructions or her role as RN. In her incident report, she wrote as a bystander in a public setting rather than an on-duty nurse at a hospital. A similar thing happened to the IEN who wrote the next piece.

CELBAN WRITING

WEEK SIX - EXAMPLE - CHOOSE YOUR LOCATION

Incident: A 65 year old man found on the floor by the elevator with an IV pole.

August 10, 2008 11:45 am. A 65 year old male fall down on the floor beside his wheelchair near the elevator with IV line intact. Pt was alone, conscious with vital signs of BP 120/80, RR 18, PR
25. Patient claims pain on his RT leg. Check for any bruises: he has light bruises on his elbow. Call for help. Mr. Adamsour LPN helped to apply a splint in the rt leg. Called for ambulance.

Debriefing

This IEN works in an extended care facility and wrote as an RN at such a facility, which does not have facilities for X-rays. For this reason the description is short and lacks details. Where this is acceptable, creating a situation that allows for more detail, in a hospital would be better.

The IEN also wrote that the man "fell down". How does she know this? Did she observe him fall? Did he tell her he fell? Could he have been pushed? Unless it is observed by the IEN or verbalized by a witness it is incorrect to write that he fell.

Choose the location. Remember, regardless of the work you are doing, when you write the CELBAN you are writing the report as a registered nurse! Choose a location for your report that allows you to write a detailed report.

CELBAN WRITING

WEEK SIX - EXAMPLE - AVOID ASSUMPTIONS

Incident: A 65 year old man found on the floor by the elevator with an IV pole.

Feb. 2, 2009, 12:00pm 65 year old man found beside wheel chair with IV pole, by the elevator. He was complaining of chest pain. His breathing was laboured. His vital signs were normal: Temp 34 degrees Celcius, pulse 100/min, Resp 12/mn, BP 180/100 mm/hg. Patient's skin was cool, his arm was limp. Called a co-worker to help to bring the patient back to bed with two person transfer. Head elevated,O2 started, and continuous monitoring. Informed the doctor, emergency blood work was ordered. Patient was on N.P.O. He was laying on the bed in a comfortable position. --Sign(RN)

Debriefing

At first, this IEN wrote, "Patient seemed to be fatigued." This is unclear and an assumption. Reporting requires clear documentation. She was asked, "How can you tell that a person is fatigued? What can you observe?" The IEN replied, "Cool skin and limp body." Write that, she was told.

Examples of Assumptions:

- Everything is fine.
- Breathing is normal.
- Vitals are normal.
- Using the word "seems".
- These statements are unclear and assumptions. Clear statements are followed by details of observations or actions. For example:
- Breathing is normal, add rate.
- Vitals are normal, add pulse, respiratory rate, blood pressure, temperature with units.

CELBAN WRITING

WEEK SIX - EXAMPLE - A GOOD START

Incident: A 65 year old man found on the floor by the elevator with an IV pole.

August 18, 2008 11:50am. Mr. X. 65 year old found on the floor beside his wheelchair with the seatbelt open. Assessment shows the following findings: IV line is intact; bruises on L foot; he is oriented to time place and person. Vital signs taken as follows: BP=180/80, PR=20. Patient moved back into the wheelchair with assistance of coworker. The physician was informed about the condition. Medications were given. All safety precautions were followed. First aid treatments were given. Documentation completed.

Debriefing

This is a good start, having chosen a hospital and knowing her role as an RN. There are a few holes: what is his name, what are his other vitals (Respiration Rate, Temperature), how the patient was transferred, what medicines were given and what dose, what safety precautions were followed, what treatments were given, and what documentation was completed.

After you read what you have written see if you have answered all of the questions or if what you wrote creates more questions.

Ask yourself ... does what I wrote create more questions.

CELBAN WRITING

WEEK SIX - EXAMPLE - VITAL SIGNS & MEDICINE

Incident: A 65 year old man found on the floor by the elevator with an IV pole.

On 10th August at 10 am 65 year old Mr Chang was found on the floor beside his wheelchair in front of the second floor elevator. His seat belt was opened and IV line came out. His left leg was stuck between the foot rest. He was conscious and narrated the incident that he was trying to enter the elevator and somehow his seatbelt opened and he fell down. He looked pale and his vital signs were stable. Abrasion present on his left foot. Called for assistance and put him back to the wheel chair. He became stable and cleared the abrasion site and applied some ointment. Notified the incident to the doctor on duty. Medications given as prescribed by him. Explained the safety precautions to him to make sure that his seat belt is on. ----------------------Signature R.N.

Debriefing

This IEN did a good job of describing observatories, medical interventions and followed many of the standards required of medical documentation. Yet there are some voids that need to be filled. Did you spot them? It is not enough to state that vital signs were stable, this statement needs to be followed by the blood pressure, respiratory rate, temperature, and pulse. It was good to note that medications were prescribed by the doctor, yet this statement needs to be followed with details not only of the medication but the dose. Complete reports allow for continuity in care.

CELBAN WRITING

WEEK SIX - EXAMPLE - FILL SPACES AND ADD TIME

Incident: A 65 year old man found on the floor by the elevator with an IV pole.

On July 13, 2008 at12:25 pm Jim Kim, patient from Rm 11 intensive care, was found on the floor inside the elevator beside the wheelchair with IV line. The patient had bruises on his face and he was pale. He said, "I don't want to be in the hospital any more." His vitals: BP 120/80, RR 22, Pulse 90. He complained of left leg pain.

Called for assistance. Took patient to the unit for observation. Diagnosis shows fracture of left leg. His vitals after 10 min: BP 130/90,RR 18, pulse 80. After...

Debriefing

This IEN did a better job of describing the situation without leaving holes: he has a name, vitals include respiratory rate, there is an explanation for where he is.

Writing in paragraphs, however, leaving a large space between words is not consistent with standards of medical documentation. If spaces are created they must be filled with a line across the space. Writing without spaces is better. The hanging sentence that begins with "After" says that this IEN ran out of time. Practicing the stages of writing in a timed setting will allow you to ensure that you use your time well.

CELBAN WRITING

WEEK SIX - EXAMPLE - DATE, TIME, SIGNATURE

Incident: A 6 year old girl found on the floor in the bathroom, a pool of liquid is on the floor.

Grace, a 6 year old girl came to the ER with left knee pain. She was accompanied by her mother, in a wheelchair, who stated that Grace was found on the wet floor in the bathroom. Her mother was a witness. Grace's knee was swollen and bruised. She complained of pain as a 7 on a scale of 10. Her vital signs were taken: P= 120/min, R=21/min, BP=90/60mmHg. The doctor was notified. The doctor ordered X-ray test at 10:00. Tylenol was given as per the doctor's order. She is sleeping in her mother's arms.

Debriefing

There are a few things missing with this IEN's report: date, time, signature. All are standard for documentation. Not only must this information be added, but it must be added in a way to ensure correct documentation procedure: without any spaces. Spaces must be filled with a line so that others may not change or add to what is written. Where the information presented is good, there are some errors. It is acceptable to include medication, as ordered by a doctor, but the dose of the medication must be included. Also, a time was given for the appointment, but it is not noted if it is in the morning or evening.

One gross error was in understanding. This assignment was for an Incident Report. Instead, the IEN wrote an assessment form. An Incident Report is required of incidents or events happening within the facility. An Assessment Report is completed when a patient is admitted to emergency, a hospital, or a clinic.

CELBAN WRITING

WEEK SIX - EXAMPLE - AVOID FIRST PERSON

Incident: A 6 year old girl found on the floor in the bathroom, a pool of liquid is on the floor.

03-09-2009 On 3rd Sept at 10 am during my morning rounds I couldn't find Misty, a 6 year old girl in her bed. When I looked in the washroom I found her on the floor. She was unconscious, breathing was shallow. I could smell some oil; the floor was wet. Physical examination done.
No bruises or discolouration found on her body. Vital signs were checked. BP was low, ie. 90/60mm of Hg. Pulse 80/mt, Resp 16/mt. I called for assistance. We put her back on her bed and immediately started oxygen. Notified the physician on duty. Medications given as advised.
Checked vital signs again. It was quite normal. She became conscious after a few minutes. Notified housekeeping for cleaning the wet floor. Sign. R.N

Debriefing

This IEN envisioned a different situation for the 6-year-old girl. As long as the situation fits and sounds reasonable any description is acceptable. Here observations were used: visual cues of a wet floor, olfactory cues of the smell of oil. Housekeeping was called in to clean up the spill. These are all great details. When it comes to medical information, some is missing. It is wonderful that the low blood pressure was noted as 90/60 but what were the other vitals? What medication was given, and how much? When vitals were checked again, what were they? Details like this are vital to accurate documentation. Otherwise, the IEN is making assumptions. This IEN also wrote in the first person using the word "I" and "We".

CELBAN WRITING

WEEK SIX - EXAMPLE - CHECK GRAMMAR

Incident: A 6 year old girl found on the floor in the bathroom, a pool of liquid is on the floor.

Sept 3, 2009 11:00 am. I answered a call from the Room 205. I found Diane, a patient, who is6 years old, on the floor. She was conscious. She was screamingand crying. Her mother Sarah said to me, "Diane was in the shower while I went to find a towel for her and she tried to go out for herself." Diane said her right hand was very painful. She answered all my questions.
Vital signs: BP 130/80, PR 130 per minute, RR: 30. Her hand is swollen and red. She can not move it. I called her paediatrician, Dr. Lung, and he ordered a X-ray of her hand and gave her acetaminaphrine 250mg tablets. She was moved to X-ray in a wheelchair. ------signature R.N.

Debriefing

The documentation of the conversation with the mother ensured that this IEN did not make any assumptions. Her description of the situation was clear and well defined. Medication was named, and the dose documented.
However, this IEN repeatedly used the word "I". In each situation, due to the medical situation and the signature, it would be appropriate to drop this word and start the sentence with the action words (Answered, Found, Called).
It is important in all writing situations to ensure that the tense of the action verb is consistent. In this piece the writer goes from past (was, said, answered) to present (is, can not). In a nursing context it s best to remain in the past tense, as the report is written after the events occurred.

CELBAN WRITING

WEEK SIX - EXAMPLE - A COMPLETE REPORT

Incident: A 6 year old girl found on the floor in the bathroom, a pool of liquid is on the floor.

4:00pm. Saturday Nov 12, 2009. 6 year old female patient found on the floor by the sink. There was wet floor, no smell and colour. She was unconscious and not able to move. Her temperature 35 degrees C, pulse 92, Resp 12, BP 90/60 mm Hg. Head to toe assessment showed back of the head had a bump, no other bruises and no skin lacerations. She was not responding. Called for assistance to bring the patient back to bed with controlled mobility and two person transfer. Start O2 and IV fluids. N.P.O and hourly observations charted. Informed doctor. Patient was dry, clean and in a comfortable position. Incident report completed by ----------------------signature R.N.

Debriefing

This Incident Report was completed by an IEN that practiced all of the stages of writing: prewriting, writing, editing and rewriting. She used the flow chart to organize her thoughts so that she included the patient information, assessment, medical intervention, charting, and evaluation.

- Can you see the difference?
- Can you tell it was written by an IEN or does it seem like a native speaker wrote this?

CELBAN WRITING

WEEK SIX - SELF-EVALUATION

How do I review my own report?

The better you get at identifying errors in the reports you write, or those written by others, the better you will get at identifying your own when editing: thus increasing your score.

To evaluate your own work, or the work of others look for the following:

- **timing:** 2 minutes mind mapping, 5 minutes writing, 5 minutes editing, 5 minutes rewriting
- spelling, punctuation, capitalization
- **grammar:** tenses consistent in the past
- **grammar:** subject-verb agreement
- reporting or charting?
- appropriate location?
- date, time, signature?
- role as an RN?
- vital signs?
- any assumptions?
- if medicine is noted, is there a dose?
- spaces filled with a line?
- a line between the report and signature?
- avoiding first person: I, me, my, we?
- integrate feedback?

Use this list to review incident reports you wrote.

WEEK SIX - YOUR TURN #1

A 16 year old man fell down on the ground near the hand sanitizer station.

Vital signs taken. BP 100/60, RR 18, PR 80. He was pail and also found bruises on his left face as caused by his fall. He verbalized that he felt dizzy and fell down. He was given water to cool him down and fresh air to breath. He said he felt better after drinking the water. Medical help came in. He was transferred on a wheel chair.

CELBAN WRITING

WEEK SIX - EVALUATON #1

Did you identify the following?

- no date, time, signature
- vitals included: good
- not assuming, adding verbalization of patient.
- not the perspective of an RN: not enough medical intervention
- no documentation
- needs more attention to using the Incident Report Flow Chart.

Take some time to re-write this report.
What would you add? What would you change?

How did you do?

The most important thing for you to do,
to increase your score.
is to be able to spot errors in your writing
and correct them.
Learn how to see your mistakes
and correct them too.

WEEK SIX - YOUR TURN #2

A 16 year old man fell down on the ground near the hand sanitizer station.

May 6, 2009 10:00 am, Mr X, 16 year old male was found in the floor near the sanitizer. He was slipped on the sanitizer. Pt was conscious but little tensed. Vitals checked. BP 140/80, HR 90, RR
26. Pt's condition was not bad. Called for assistance. With help of two other people shifted the patient to the bed. Informed the patient's condition to the doctor on duty. Checked the patient for any injuries. There was slight bruises in both legs and in the left
arm. Patient complaints of pain. Analgesics given as ordered by the doctor. Checked for head injuries: nothing found. Dressing done on
the wound. --------------------- ------------------signature RN
12:00pm. Vitals checked again. It was normal. Now patient looks
better. -- signRN

CELBAN WRITING

WEEK SIX - EVALUATON #3

Did you identify the following?

By now you should see a common error:

- "seems unstable",
- "seems stable"
- "feels relief".

These three statements are assumptions that need clarification.

Also:

- Vitals were not documented.
- A question also arises, how did this IEN know what happened? It is not documented that the patient told her what happened.
- Furthermore, how could "I reported to the doctor" be reworded to eliminate the word "I"?

WEEK SIX - YOUR TURN #3

A 16 year old man fell down on the ground near the hand sanitizer station.

On May 3rd 2009, at 10:00 am, 16 year old boy found on the ground near to the sanitizer. He was trying to reach to the sanitizer but unable to reach. His foot got stuck on his wheel chair and fell down. He had redness and bruises on his right foot and left arm.
His vitals was taken but it seems unstable. Call for help and two person transfer to the wheelchair. I reported to the doctor. All the precript medicine given and applied some ointment on his injured part. After a few minutes his vitals seems stable and he feels relief. -------------signature RN

CELBAN WRITING

WEEK SIX - EVALUATON #2

Did you identify the following?

- include date, time signature
- fill in spaces
- no name of patient
- correct use of additional entry
- appropriate use of abbreviation ` "Pt"
- incomplete information: analgesic given
- grammar: preposition "in"
- grammar: verb, "was slipped"
- grammar: subject-verb agreement, "was bruises"
- grammar: using noun instead of verb, "patient complaints"

This wording needs details to add clarity and clarify assumptions:

- patient was little tense,
- patient complains of pain,
- vitals normal,
- patient looks better.

CELBAN WRITING

WEEK SIX - ASSIGNMENT

Using the Incident Flow Chart, your assignment is to write an incident report.

Follow the steps:

- **5 min** writing, and
- **5 min** editing,

1. Having completed the pre-writing stage, in the previous lesson, you are ready to write your work. Using a timer, practice writing your incident report.
2. In five minutes or less, edit the incident report you have written. When you have completed this step go on to the next step.
3. Having completed the editing stage, rewrite the report, in less than five minutes.
4. Using the flow charts you created, spend at least half an hour a day writing an incident report, using your work from last week.

Practice the process of transforming your completed incident report flow charts into written incident reports. This time instead of doing one step at a time, you will do all of the stages at once.

Week Seven

CELBAN WRITING

WEEK SEVEN - MEDICAL HISTORIES

Can I use this process to write other types of medical reports?

YES!

You can apply the stages of writing to anything you write. But, just to prove the point, we will now explore using the stages of writing to write a report about a patient's medical history using a similar but different flow chart to get you started.

Previously, for Prewriting, you were encouraged to brainstorm a mind map of ideas from which you would create your paragraph on a certain topic related to writing an incident report. For the writing component of the CELBAN, the topics are related to documentation in a nursing context. For the previous lesson, we explored writing Incident Reports. For this lesson, you will apply the same transferable skills to taking a patient's medical history. In doing so you will also be preparing for speaking and listening tasks.

- What are some of the elements that go into an assessment report?
- What is the first thing you ask a patient?

Right, you ask for personal information. You might also ask about the patient's lifestyle. Next, you would ask about symptoms. With this information, you might provide medical intervention. To conclude the assessment, you would complete some sort of documentation.

These are the essential elements of an assessment report.

CELBAN WRITING

WEEK SEVEN - FLOW CHART

How is an Assessment Flow Chart different from an Incident Report Flow Chart?

At the point of creating a flow chart for an assessment report, the information is the same as that for the incident report.

There are five general subheadings:

- **Patient Information**: gender, age, health status and other general information
- **Lifestyle:** smoking, drinking, diet, exercise, stress etc.
- **Assessment/Symptoms:** Blood Pressure, Heart Rate, Temperature, Respiratory Rate
- **Medical Interventions:** education, medication, dressings, etc.
- **Documentation:** completion/commencement of charts and other necessary documentation

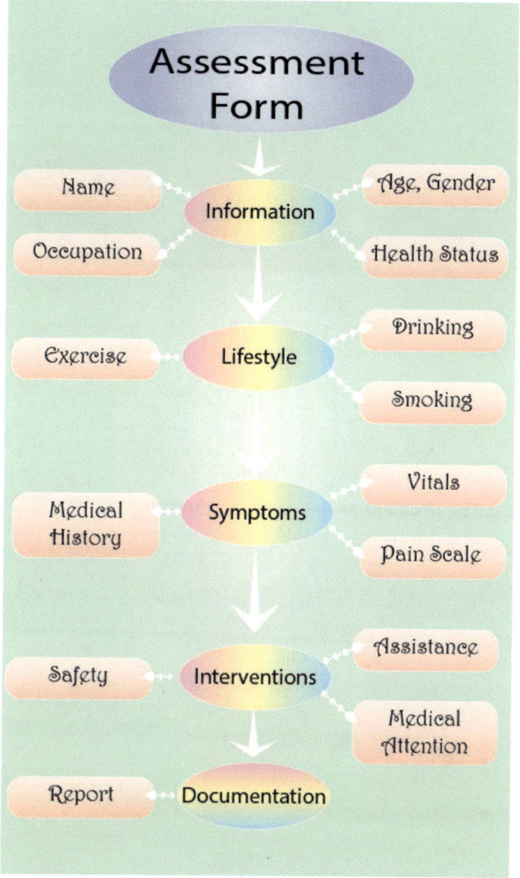

These five general subheadings make up the outline for documentation reports, and become the mind map for the Pre-Writing portion of the CELBAN.

CELBAN WRITING

WEEK SEVEN - OBSERVATIONS

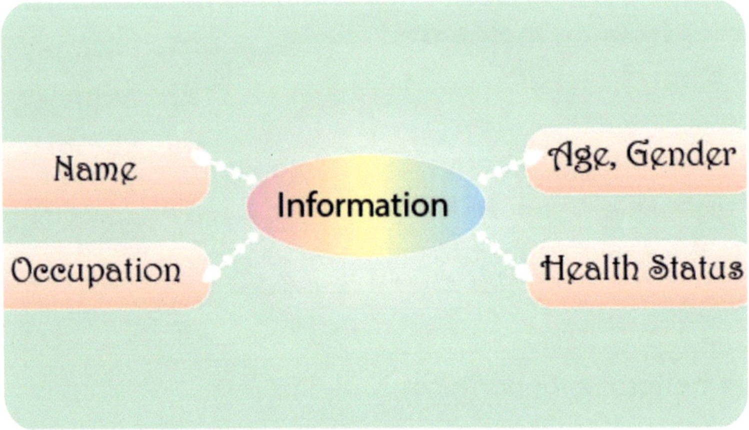

Information

What basic information do you seek as a registered nurse performing an assessment?

- Name,
- Age,
- Gender,
- Occupation, and
- Health Status.

All of these elements are components of personal information that are required.

CELBAN WRITING

WEEK SEVEN - ASSESSMENT

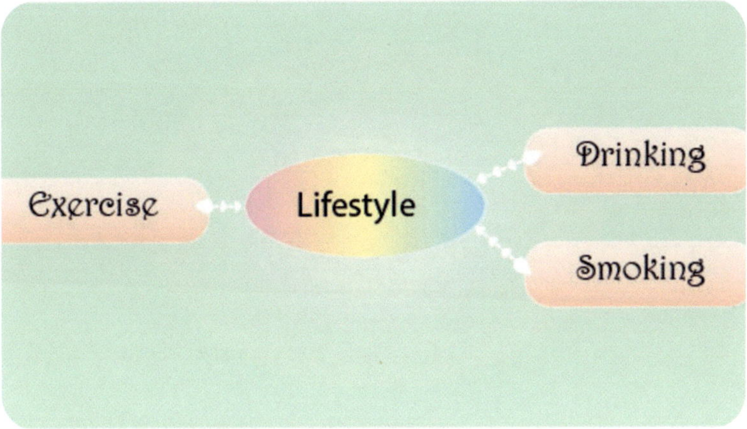

Lifestyle

When you are asking a patient about their lifestyle, what kind of questions would you ask? You would ask if the patient:

- smokes,
- drinks, or
- exercises.

What are some other elements of lifestyle?

CELBAN WRITING

WEEK SEVEN - SYMPTOMS

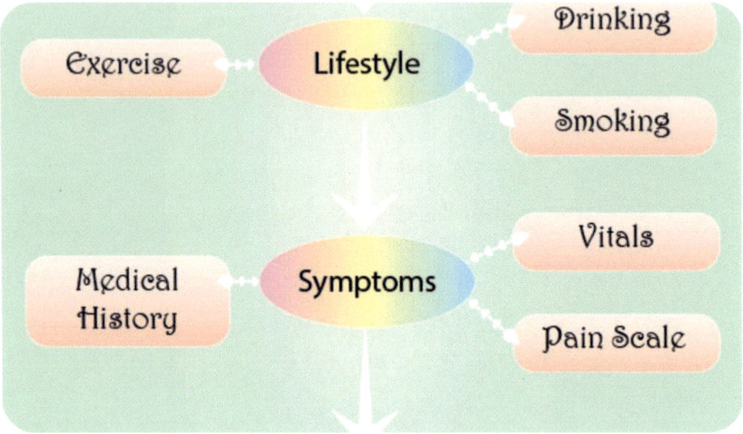

Symptoms

What do you need to know about a patient, when he or she arrives at the hospital? What kind of questions can you ask about:

- medical history,
- vitals,
- pain scale?

That is what you would add to this flow chart, in preparation for writing a report.

CELBAN WRITING

WEEK SEVEN - DOCUMENTATION

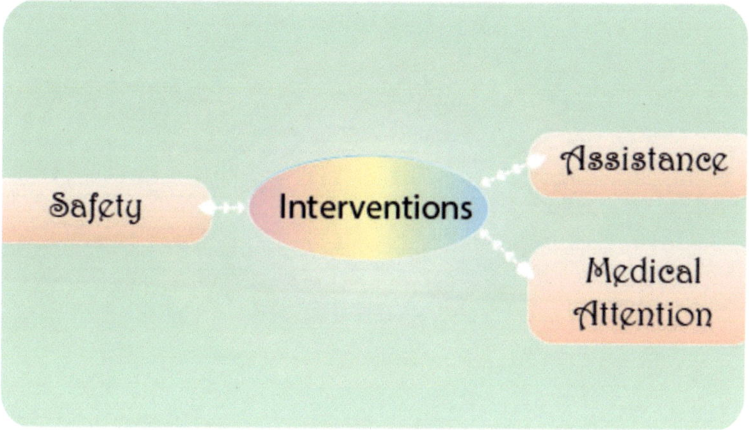

Interventions

Whether you are conducting an assessment after an incident or upon arrival at the clinic, as a licensed nurse, the process of gathering information is the same. So is the writing of medical intervention and documentation. What can you write about:

- ensuring patient safety,
- getting or giving assistance,
- providing medical attention?

CELBAN WRITING

WEEK SEVEN - DOCUMENTATION

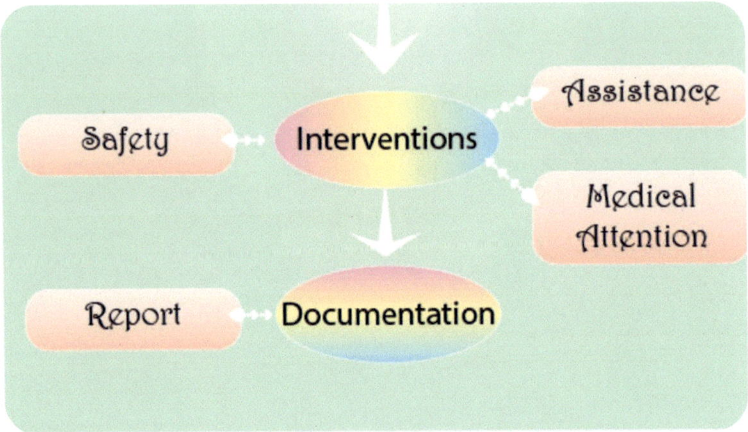

Documentation

In a medical context, documentation is documentation. Little does it vary. Forms and policies are created, used and upheld. Similar to the incident report, there are several other documentation processes that can be included in a patient assessment report. This includes but is not limited to the following:

- beginning a blood sugar chart,
- charting continuous monitoring,
- hourly observations,
- input/output and
- pleur- evac chart.

What other kinds of reports or charts would you use?

CELBAN WRITING

WEEK SEVEN - FLOW CHART

How do I put the pieces together?

Thus, a Medical Assessment Flow Chart, based on an Assessment Form, can be used as the basis for pre-writing. All it takes is adding more details.

On the next two pages, you will see an Assessment Flow chart with patient details added. Use these details to write your own report. Remember the guidance that was provided in the previous lesson when it comes to:

- location,
- dates and times,
- avoiding "I" statements,
- avoiding assumptions,
- including your role as the medical professional,
- checking grammar, punctuation, capitalization, and sentence structure.

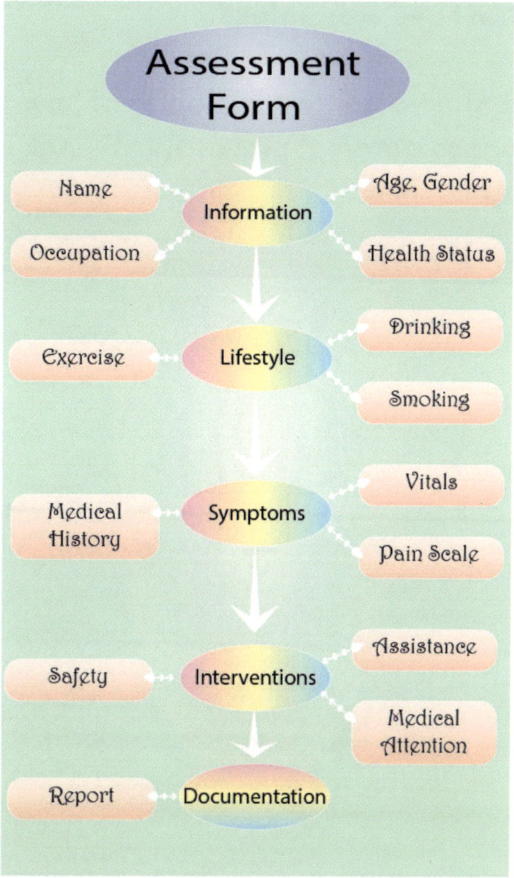

Remember to time your self:

- 5 minutes to write, and
- 5 minutes to edit.

CELBAN WRITING

WEEK SEVEN - MEDICAL HISTORIES

Can I see examples?

YES! Here are two examples of how the Assessment Form flow chart was used for two different patients. Let's look at them one at a time, so you can write a report.

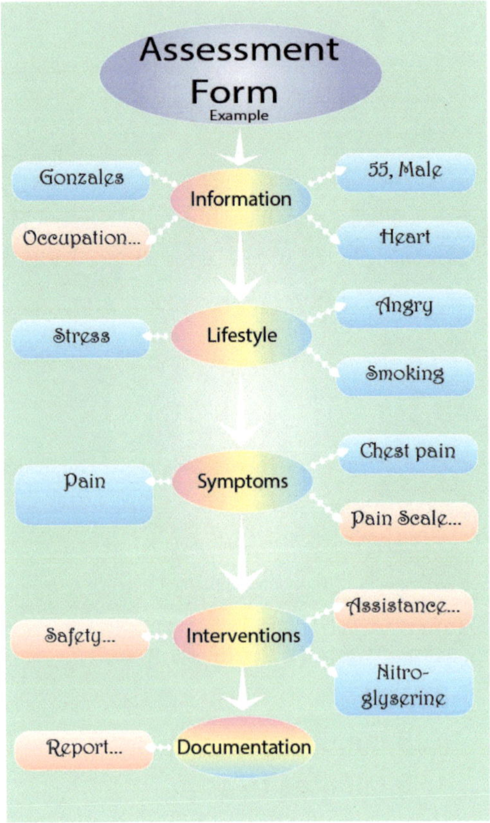

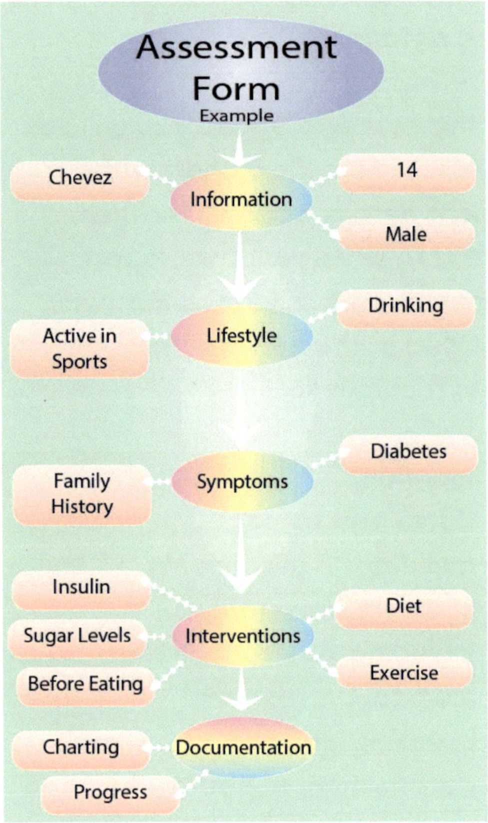

CELBAN WRITING

WEEK SEVEN - YOUR TURN #1

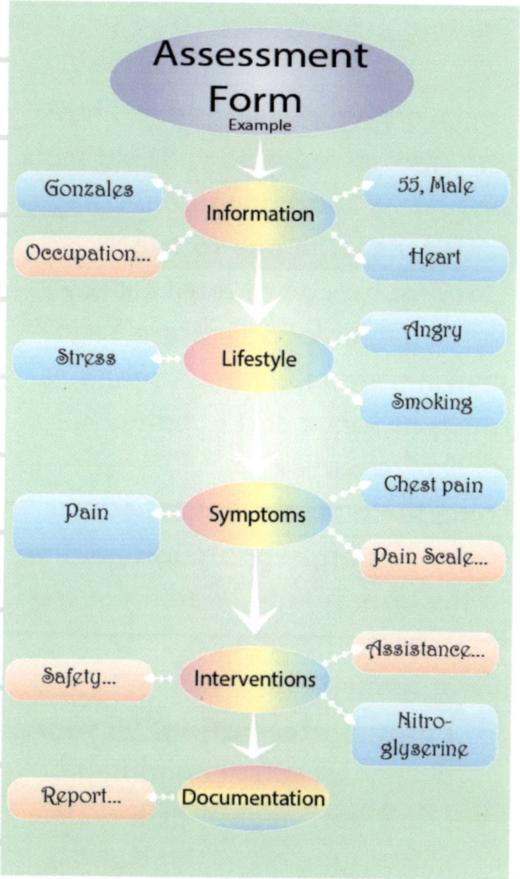

Remember to time your self:

- Mind mapping has been done.
- 5 minutes to write, and
- 5 minutes to edit.

CELBAN WRITING

WEEK SEVEN - THINKING PROCESS

How do I do this?

Thinking process

I am working in emergency. I have just interviewed a 55 year old male who has a heart condition. Using sentences write one to two paragraphs. Use at least six key words: high blood pressure, smoking, stress, nitro-glycerine, family history, heart conditions, alcohol, exercise

Using the 6 points above I can assign the appropriate information to the appropriate heading of the flow chart. This can be done in linear form:

- **Patient Information:** 55 year old, male, health condition
- **LifeStyle:** smoker, history of chest pain, angry, high stress
- **Assessment/Symptoms:** high cholesterol, chest pains, angry
- **Medical Intervention:** nitroglycerine
- **Documentation:** report

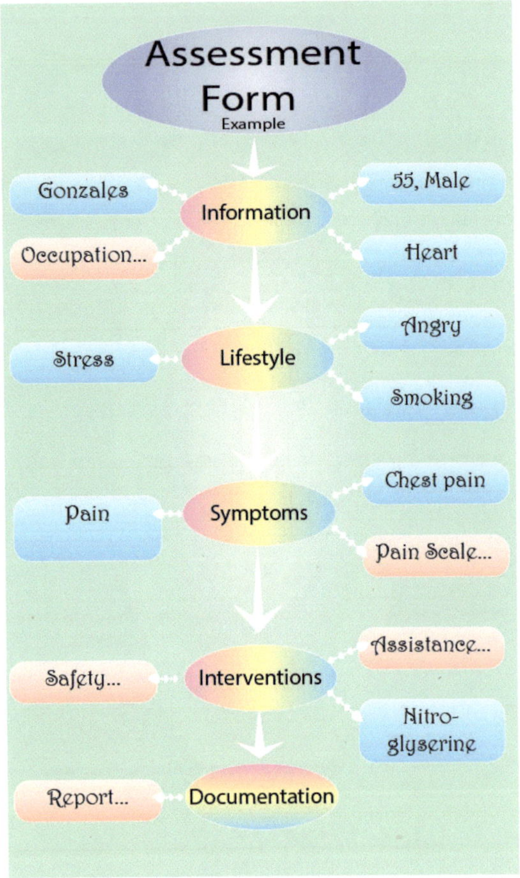

CELBAN WRITING

WEEK SEVEN - EXAMPLE REPORT

Time: 10 pm
Date: January 24, 2009

55 year old male interviewed in the emergencyroom. He was worried about his health condition. His job was stressful. Companylayed him off.
he had a history of has heart attach. Patient cholesterol level was high. and he gets angery very quickly. Whenever hte doctor perscribed the medication nytroglycerins. his vital signs was abnormal. Nitroglycerine given. continuous
montitoring. Informed the doctor and emergency blood work done. Hea was a heavy smoker. He was lived in a stressful condition. Assessment completed by

signature.

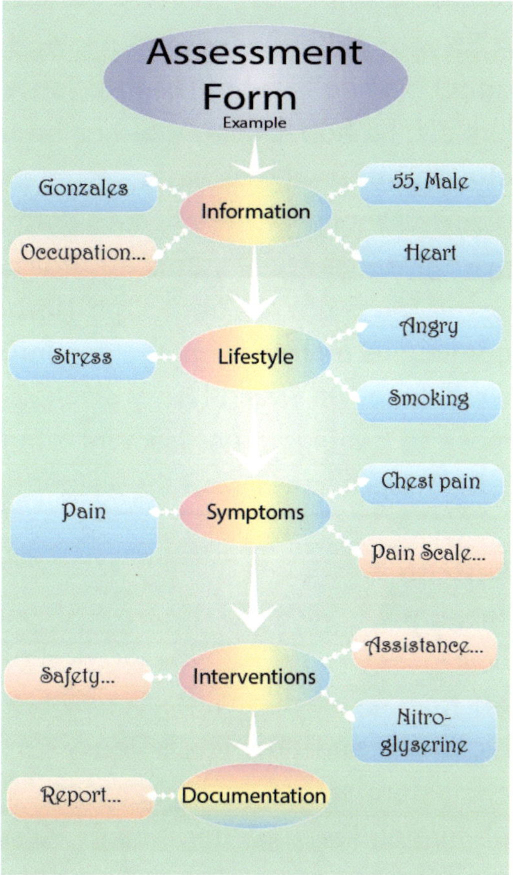

It is easy to see in reading this assessment that the flow chart was used to ensure that all of the information was included.

CELBAN WRITING

WEEK EVEN - EXAMPLE - EDIT

Time: 10 pm fix
Date: January 24, 2009
delete space
A 55 year old male was interviewed in the emergency room. He was worried about his health condition. His job was stressful. Company layed spelling him off. he had a history of has heart attach. Delete and re-write Patient cholesterol level was high. delete period and he gets angery spelling very quickly. Whenever hte spelling doctor perscribed spelling the medication nytroglycerins spelling. his capitalize vital signs was abnormal. add more detail: what are the vital signs Nitroglycerine given. capitalize and fix continuous montitoring. spelling Informed the doctor and emergency blood work done. He was a heavy smoker. He was lived in a stressful condition. move to beginning Assessment completed by not necessary
add line and move signature signature

Rewrite

January 24, 2009, 10:00pm. A 55 year old male was interviewed in the emergency room. He was worried about his health condition; he was laid off from his company. His family history includes heart conditions and high blood pressure. He was a heavy smoker; he lived in a stressful condition. His cholesterol level was high; he could not control his anger. His vital signs was abnormal: Temp 35 degrees C, Pulse 100/min, Resp 12/min, B.P. 180/120 mm/ Hg. the patient's head was elevated,O2 was started, nitroglycerin was given, and continuous monitoring charted. -------------------------------------

The doctor was informed; emergency blood work was done. -------Sign RN

CELBAN WRITING

WEEK SEVEN - DEBRIEFING

I can do that?
YES! You can! What a remarkable improvement! Can you see the difference that organization, good punctuation, proper spelling and grammar make? That is what makes the writing steps of editing and re-writing so valuable.

That is the value of the CELBANPrep Suite:

- **CELBAN Writing Preparation Guide, and**
- **the *Grammar Essentials*!**

With practice, this Internationally Educated Nurse was able to write a nursing context paragraph within the 15 minutes given during the CELBAN. By the time she wrote the CELBAN, she was able to organize her thoughts in seconds, allowing plenty of time to write, edit, and re-write!

Editing in the Nursing Context, for the CELBAN, requires reviewing one's own writing for spelling, punctuation, grammar, and organization. Common grammar errors for Internationally Educated Nurses include:

- **Verb tense:** using both present and past tense
- **Single/Plural Agreement:** using a single noun with a plural verb or a plural noun with a singular verb (he were, they was)
- Confusing **pronouns** (you, he, she) with possessives (yours, his, hers)
- **Prepositions**: (in, at, on)
- **Articles** (a, an, the)

CELBAN WRITING

WEEK SEVEN - YOUR TURN #2

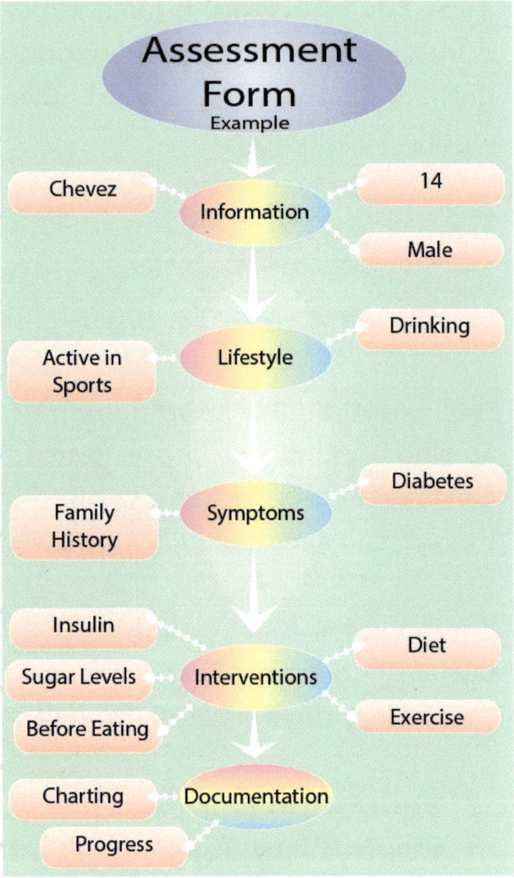

Remember to time your self:

- Mind mapping has been done.
- 5 minutes to write, and
- 5 minutes to edit.

CELBAN WRITING

WEEK SEVEN - THINKING PROCESS

How do I do this?

I am working in a clinic. I just completed an interview with a 14 year old male. Using complete sentences I will write 1-2 paragraphs describing the patient's situation.

I will use six of the following words: diabetes, insulin, blood sugar level, needle, diet, sugar, obesity, exercise.

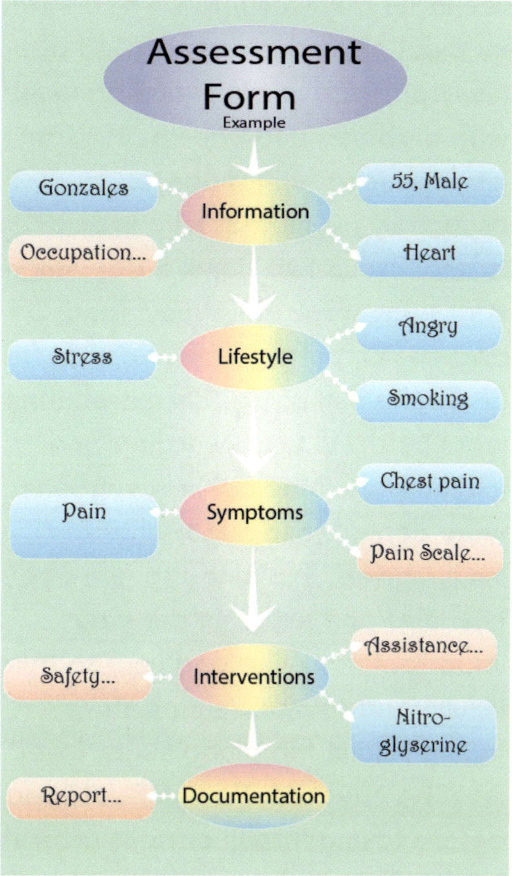

CELBAN WRITING

WEEK SEVEN - EXAMPLE REPORT

Sept 25, 2009, 3:45 pm. 14 year old teenager boy was interviewed in the medical clinic. He was worried about his health status. He was diagnosed with diabetes and obesity. His family history shows high diabetes, especially his mother who is also taking insulin two times a day. His vital signs were abnormal: Temp 34 degrees C, pulse 60/mt, Resp 14/mt, BP 80/50 mm of Hg. His extremities were cold. He was sweating and looked pale. Medical Interventions were done: blood sugar checked, insulin given. Explained to him about how diet and exercise are very important in his life and how to take insulin and to make sure before taking insulin the blood sugar level must be checked. He must eat food before taking insulin or right after the insulin. The doctor was informed. Blood Sugar chart was maintained. ------signature

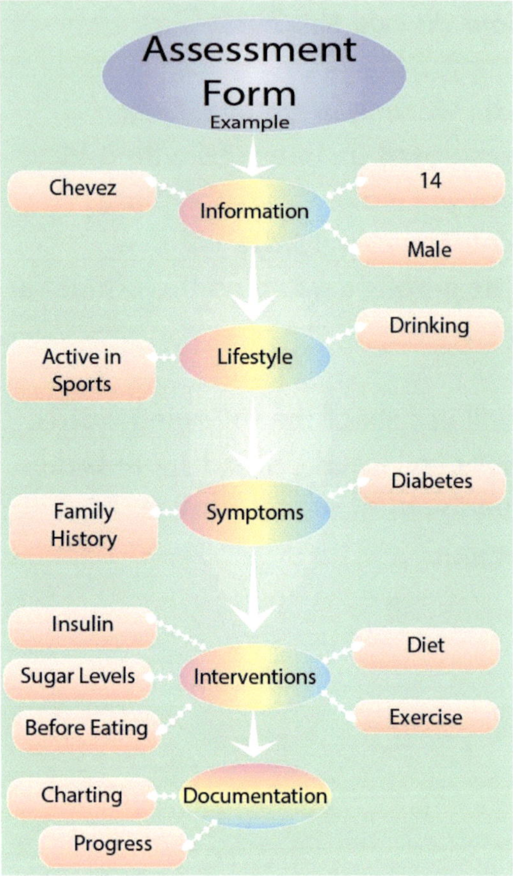

It is easy to see in reading this assessment that the flow chart was used to ensure that all of the information was included.

CELBAN WRITING

WEEK SEVEN - ASSIGNMENT

How do I apply this to my own writing?

This lesson's assignment is similar to the one for incident reports, except that information is given for you to add to the assessment. You have to choose key terms from a list, and use them in your report.

For this assignment you apply everything you have learned before: stages of writing, timing yourself, editing, ensuring you are following medical documentation standards. As a result, your assignment should be error-free: at least with very few errors.

Make sure you take the time to edit your report: spot errors and correct them to increase your score. You must be able to self-correct grammar, spelling, punctuation, and capitals for this lesson.

Here is an example:

- You are working at an extended care facility. You have just interviewed a 72-year-old male who has Alzheimer's. Using sentences, write one to two paragraphs. Use at least six keywords: memory loss, walking, incontinence, anger, aggressive, bruise, eating, medicine, urine check.

While an assessment report is not part of CELBAN writing, conducting a patient history in CELBAN speaking is. So writing these reports helps you prepare for that.

CELBAN WRITING

WEEK SEVEN - FLOW CHART ASSIGNMENT

Combine the Stages of Writing and the Assessment Report Flow Chart to write reports.

- Spend at least 30 minutes a day writing assessment reports.
- Use the list of situations you brainstormed earlier.
- Using the stages of writing practice in a timed setting.
- Using the information organized during the pre-writing stage
- Include relevant details
- Add the time and the date
- Remember to add a line at the bottom of the text with your signature, as standard nursing practice.
- Include what you have learned through grammar resources to the editing stage.
- Include what you learned about writing incident reports in the lesson and from feedback you received with your CELBAN results.

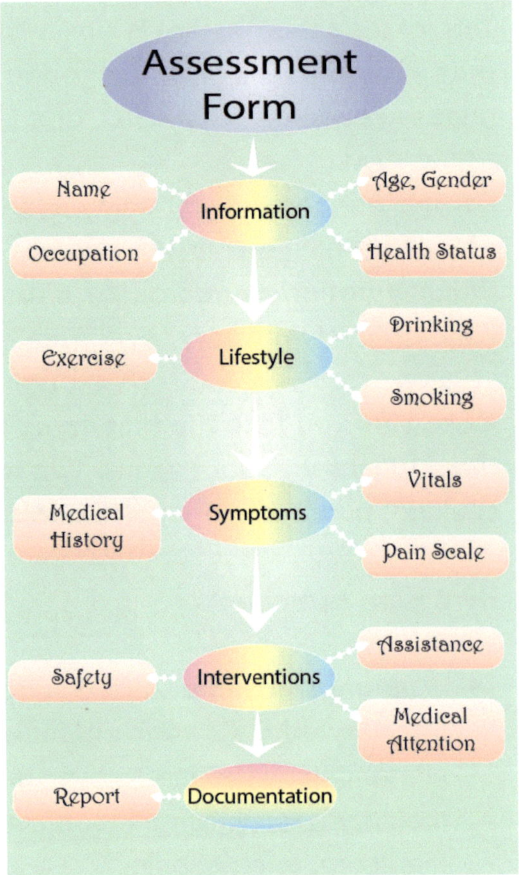

Remember to time your self:

- 2 minutes to mind map,
- 5 minutes to write, and
- 5 minutes to edit.

CELBAN WRITING

WEEK SEVEN - SELF EVALUATION

How do I apply this to my own writing?

The better you get at identifying errors in the reports you write, or those written by others, the better you will get at identifying your own when editing: thus increasing your score.

To evaluate your own work, or the work of others, look for the following:

- timing
  - **2 minutes** mind mapping,
  - **5 minutes** writing,
  - **5 minutes** editing,
- spelling, punctuation, capitalization
- grammar: tenses consistent in the past
- grammar: subject-verb agreement
- appropriate location?
- date, time, signature?
- role as an RN?
- vital signs?
- any assumptions?
- if medicine is noted, is there a dose?
- spaces filled with a line?
- a line between the report and signature?
- avoiding first person: I, me, my, we?
- include feedback?

USE THIS LIST TO REVIEW ASSESSMENT REPORTS YOU HAVE WRITTEN

HAVING TROUBLE CREATING SENTENCES?

Use these dictionaries to find common phases used in medical contexts and situations.

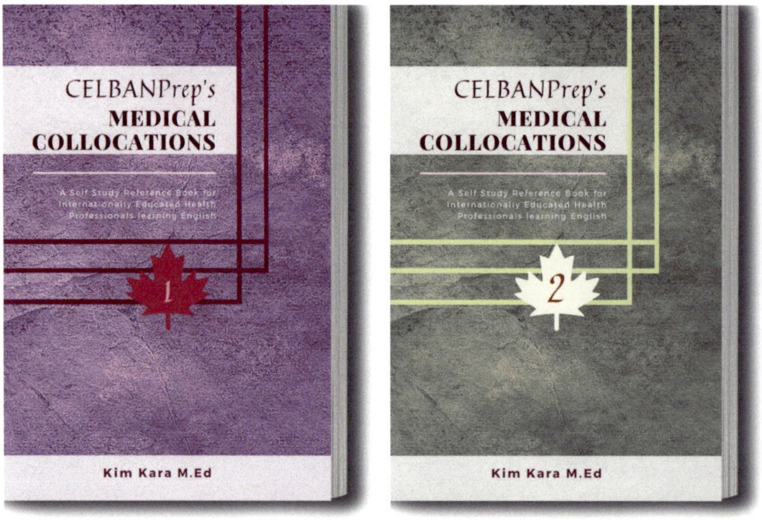

UNLOCK THE POWER OF PRECISE COMMUNICATION:

Your success in healthcare starts now!

Week Eight

NAME ______________________ **DATE** ______________________

CELBAN WRITING

HEALER CELEBRATE THY SELF

Contemplate the ROLE of CELBANPrep

Write down all the reasons ways that CELBANPrep Writing has helped you to Prepare for the CELBAN.

NAME ______________________ **DATE** ______________________

CELBAN WRITING

HEALER CELEBRATE THY SELF

Contemplate the ROLE of CELBANPrep

Think about all the different roles you play, as a nurse, with all the different contexts. **Write down a point-form list** of when and how you will apply what you have learned through CELBANPrep writing. (Avoid limiting your self to just writing.)

NAME ____________________ **DATE** ____________________

CELBAN WRITING

HEALER CELEBRATE THY SELF

Contemplate the ROLE of CELBANPrep

Imagine your life, now and in the future, as a result of preparing for the CELBAN through CELBANPrep writing. What do you see for your self when it comes to your dreams, your aspirations, your future.

NAME ____________________ **DATE** ____________________

CELBAN WRITING

HEALER CELEBRATE THY SELF

Contemplate the ROLE of CELBANPrep

Expand upon what you wrote on the last page by including your well being: emotionally, mentally, physically and spiritually.

NAME ______________________ **DATE** ______________________

CELBAN WRITING

HEALER CELEBRATE THY SELF

Contemplate the ROLE of CELBANPrep

What has happened to your level of confidence and motivation the past 8 weeks while you have embarked on preparing for the CELBAN through CELBANPrep?

NAME ______________________ **DATE** ______________________

CELBAN WRITING

HEALER CELEBRATE THY SELF

Contemplate the ROLE of CELBANPrep

What has been the most valuable aspect of CELBANPrep Writing?

NAME ______________________ **DATE** ______________________

CELBAN WRITING

HEALER CELEBRATE THY SELF

Contemplate the ROLE of CELBANPrep

What will you tell your friends?

NAME ____________________ **DATE** ____________________

CELBAN WRITING

HEALER CELEBRATE THY SELF

Contemplate the ROLE of CELBANPrep

Write a review, then share it on
Facebook, LinkedIn, Google, and/or Amazon.

Week Nine

NAME ______________________ **DATE** ______________________

______________________ ______________________

CELBAN WRITING

REFLECTIONS

People often complain that at CELBANPrep we do not teach as others do. We do not provide sample tests and practice exams. Instead, we provide ample reflection to create a solid foundation for your studies, then we provide activities where you can increase your skills and competencies: at home, at work and in the community. And we teach you how to create your own questions so that you never run out!

What have you learned about your own learning process and the effectiveness of this method of instruction?

NAME ______________________ **DATE** ______________________

What have you learned about your own ability to create your own questions?

NAME ____________________ **DATE** ____________________

How has this been helpful not only for your preparations for the CELBAN but also life in general?

Please share what you learned, and how your perceptions have changed, as a review on Amazon not only for writing but also the other 3 skills.

CELBAN WRITING PREPARATION GUIDE

Congratulations

Created by CELBANPrep University
Published by CELBANPrep Publishing

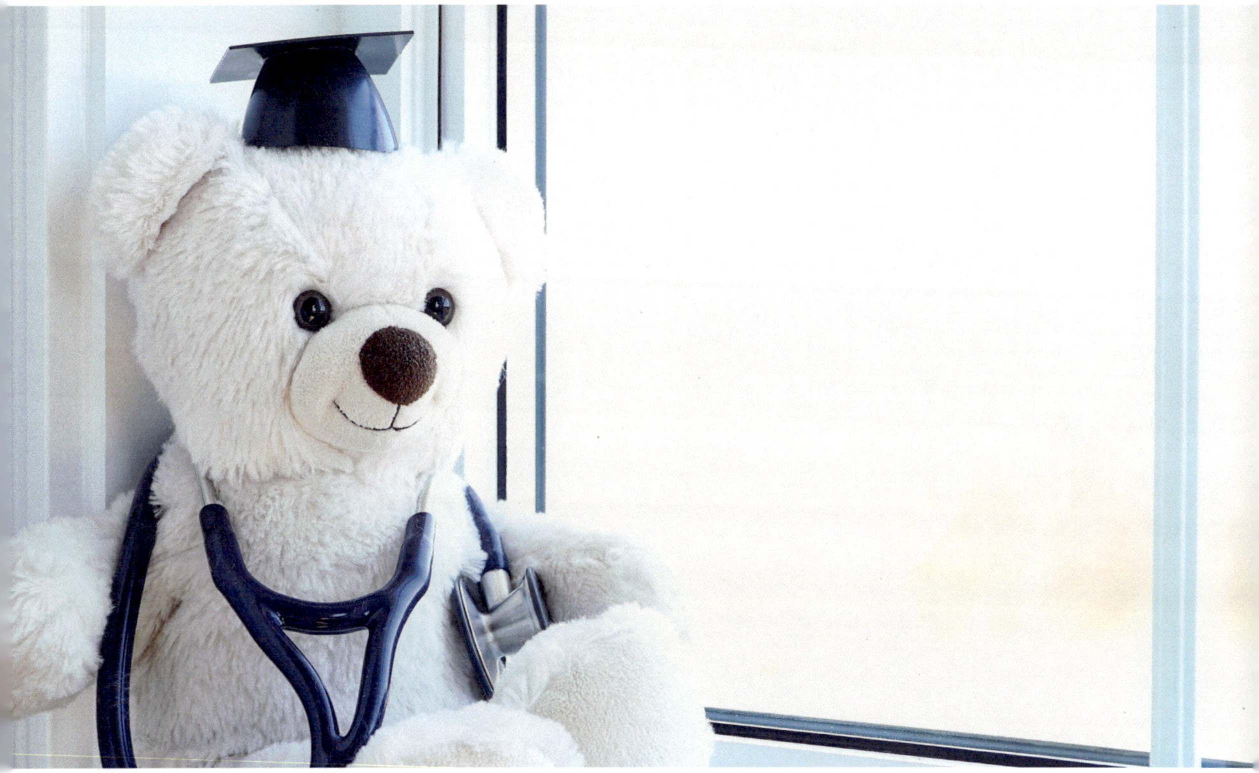

YOU HAVE COMPLETED CELBANPREP WRITING LEVEL TWO

Pause to Contemplate Your Journey

YOU MIGHT LIKE

E-BOOK AVAILABLE INTERNATIONALLY ON AMAZON

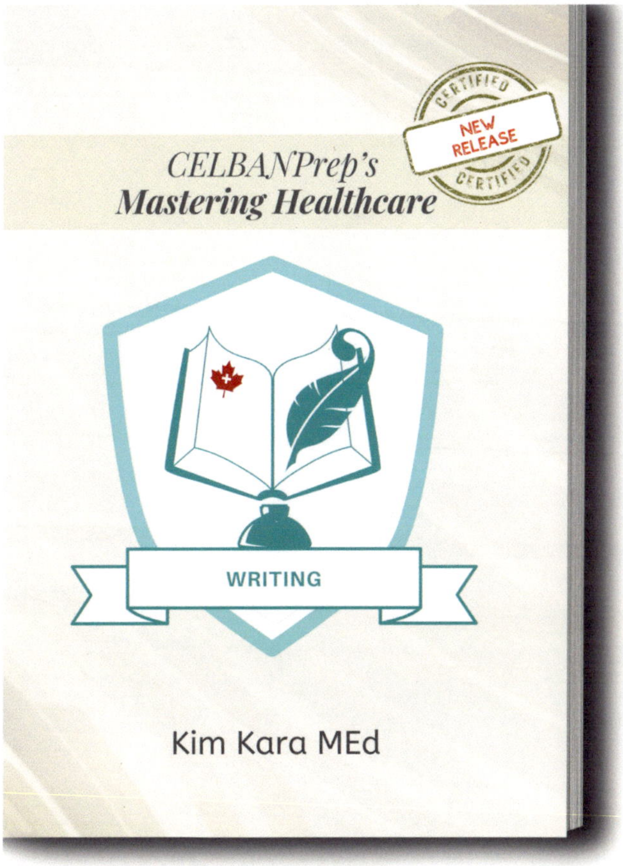

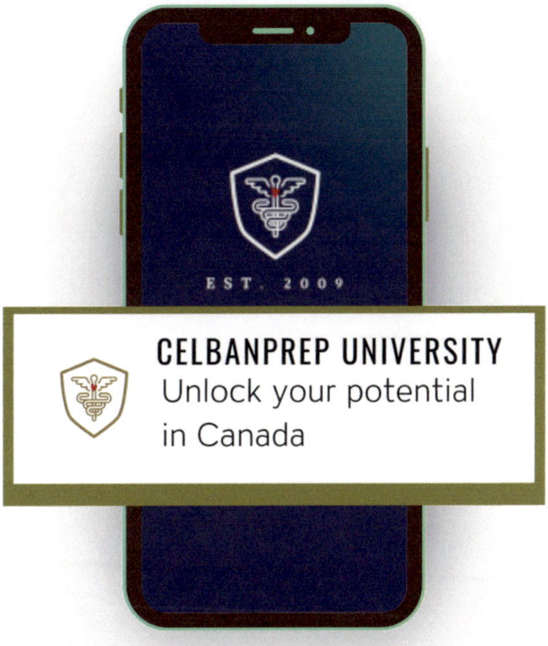

ENGLISH LANGUAGE MASTERY

FOR HEALTH PROFESSIONALS

Made in the USA
Las Vegas, NV
03 November 2026

57423450R00124